Understanding Heart Disease
A Guide For Patients And Their Families

Understanding Heart Disease
A Guide For Patients And Their Families

John Durand, M.D., F.A.C.C.

Mockingbird Communications

Notice:

This book is not a substitute for medical care provided by your own doctor. No two cases are the same, and this book is in no manner intended to replace, countermand or conflict with the advice of your own doctor. Keep your doctor informed of your condition, since only your physician can diagnose and treat a medical problem.

To my beloved wife and friend Susie, for her understanding and acceptance of my ways, and to our son Jeff, who is the joy of our lives.

Contents

Angina

Chapter 5   **89**

Preparing for Recovery and Hospital Discharge

Chapter 6   **107**

Artery and Vein Disorders

Illustrations & Tables

Preface

Perhaps you or a family member has recently been diagnosed as having a heart or blood vessel disorder. The goal of this book is to provide you with a better understanding of heart disease, its treatment, and its prevention. Not every chapter will apply to your case, so choose among the chapters and read at a pace that is suited best for you. At first you may want to know only a few basics about your condition, and later – as time and energy permits – you may wish to continue your reading to expand your understanding. Share this book with family and friends since they may also have questions about your condition and medical treatment.It is my hope that this book will improve your understanding of heart disease and enhance communication between you and your physician.

John Durand, M.D., F.A.C.C.

How The Heart And Circulation Work

The heart is an amazing pump which circulates 50 million gallons of blood in an average person's lifetime.Oxygen-depleted blood first enters the right side of the heart through the *right atrium* traveling through the *tricuspid valve* into the *right ventricle* (Figure I-1). The right ventricle then pumps blood through the *pulmonary valve* into the lungs where carbon dioxide is extracted and exhaled. Oxygen enters the blood through lung capillaries and oxygen-enriched blood then returns to the left-sided pumping chambers.

Here blood enters the *left atrium* and traverses the *mitral valve*, entering the main heart pumping chamber, the *left ventricle*. The left ventricle is the major working chamber of the heart performing approximately five times greater mechanical work load than any other cardiac chamber. Under high pressure, the left ventricle forcefully pumps blood through the *aortic valve* into the *aorta*.

The *arteries* then distribute oxygen-rich blood under high pressure to all body tissues (Figure I-3). Once blood enters the capillary system, oxygen is extracted, and the oxygen-depleted blood returns through a large network of draining veins. *Veins* carry blood under low pressure back toward the right side of the heart through the major veins , the *superior vena cava* and the *inferior vena cava* (Figure I-4). The cycle then repeats itself.

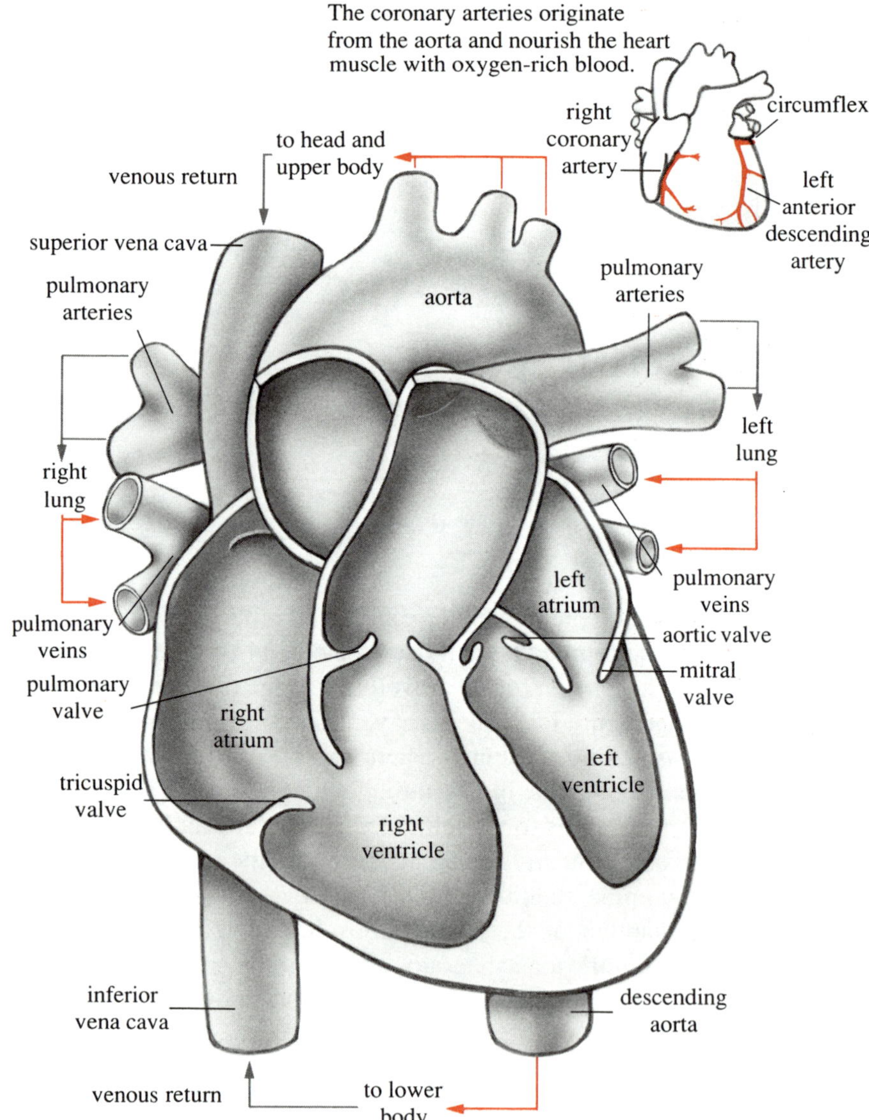

Oxygen-poor venous blood returns from the upper and lower body
to the right atrium, where it is pumped into the lungs and enriched
with oxygen. The oxygen-rich arterial blood returns to the left
ventricle and is pumped under high pressure to all body parts.
Heart valves prevent back-leakage as blood is pumped forward
through the heart chambers.

2 Understanding Heart Disease

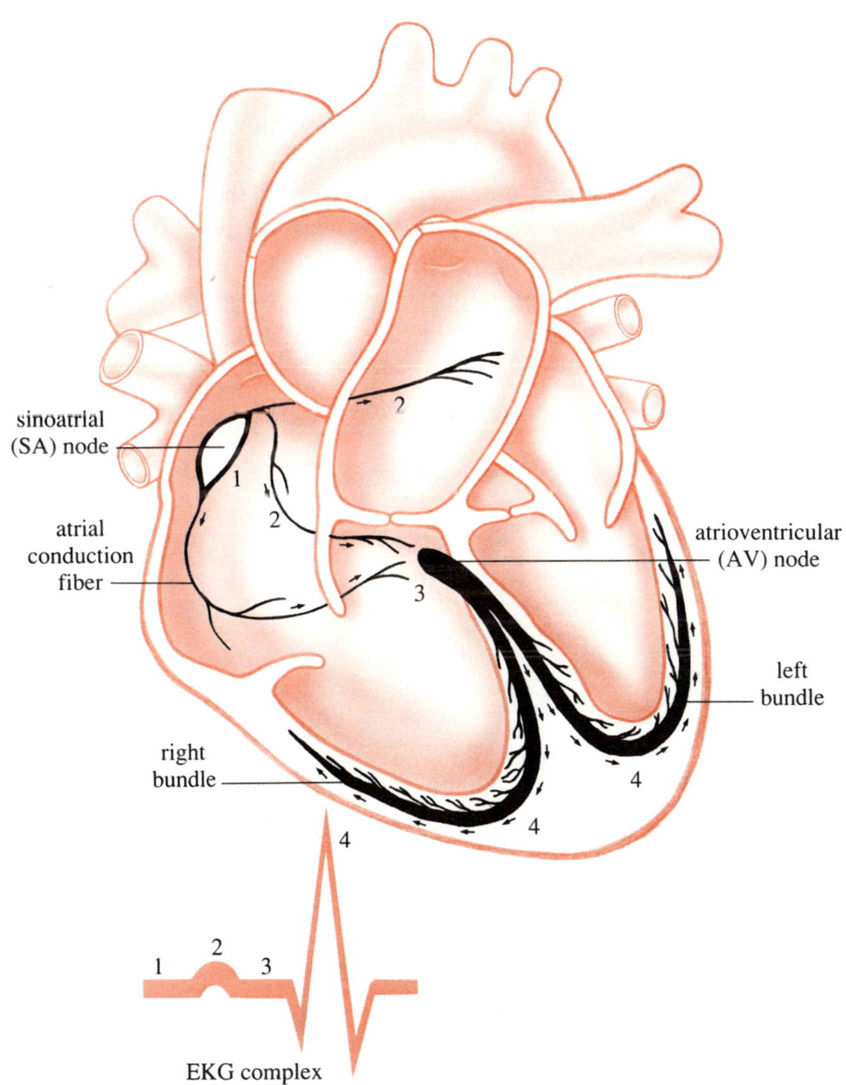

Electrical impulses originate from the SA node (1) and pass through electrical fibers (2,3,4) of the heart, generating the EKG complex.

The heart muscle requires a constant supply of nutrients in order to perform its pumping action. These nutrients are exclusively supplied by the *coronary arteries* which run on the surface of the heart. The heart does not extract nutrients from the blood within the cardiac chambers. *Valves* within the heart chambers direct blood forward, preventing back leakage of blood as the main pumping chambers contract.

The heart rhythm is controlled by a small electrical clock at the top of the heart called the *sinoatrial node* (Figure I-1). Approximately every 8/10 of a second this small electrical clock discharges its electrical activity, sending a nerve-like impulse first through the atrial chambers and then to the ventricular chambers. This causes an orderly sequence of atrial contraction followed by ventricular contraction. Disruption of this natural electrical pathway within the heart results in irregularities in heart beat termed *arrhythmia*.

Blockage in coronary blood flow can result in heart pain called *angina* or actually damage an area of heart muscle resulting in heart attack, or *myocardial infarction*.

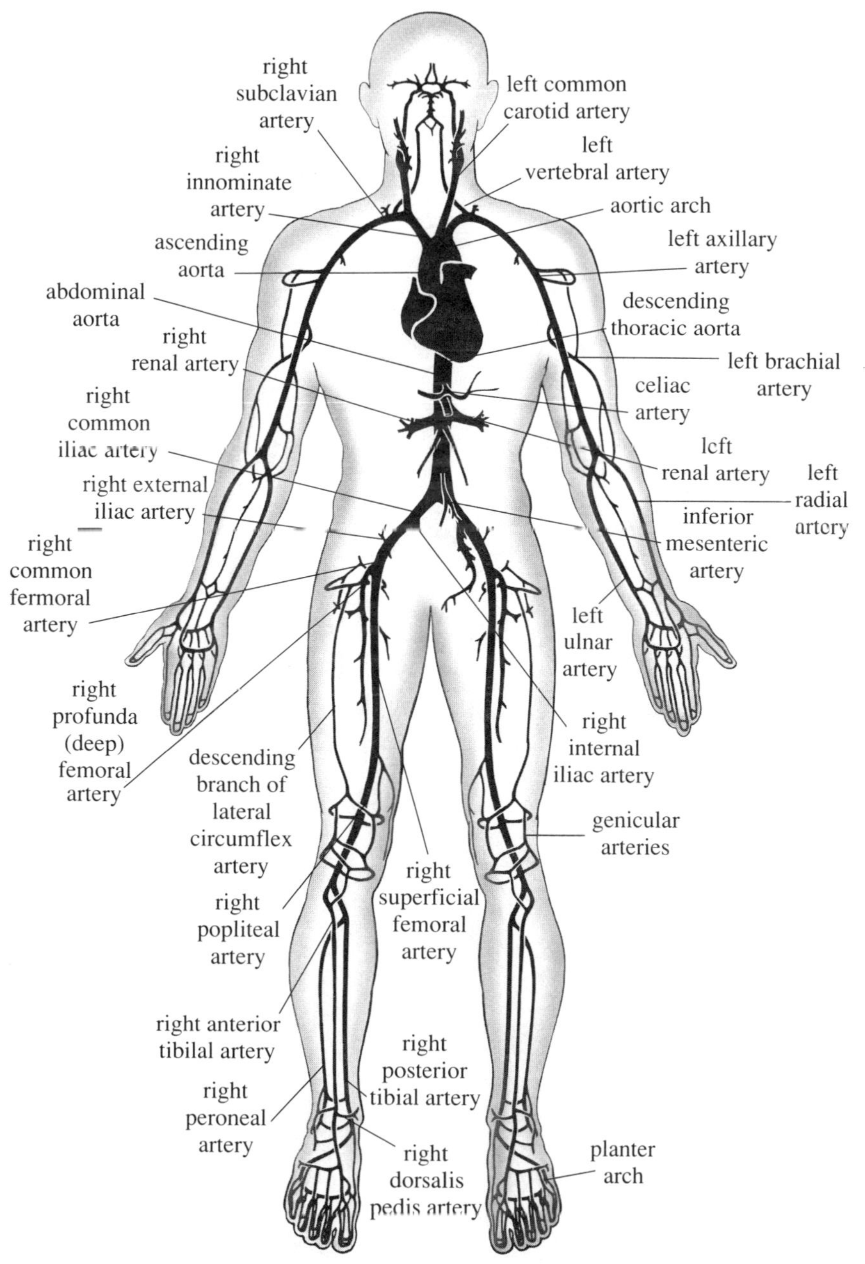

right subclavian artery
left common carotid artery
right innominate artery
left vertebral artery
aortic arch
ascending aorta
left axillary artery
abdominal aorta
descending thoracic aorta
right renal artery
left brachial artery
right common iliac artery
celiac artery
left renal artery
right external iliac artery
left radial artery
right common fermoral artery
inferior mesenteric artery
left ulnar artery
right profunda (deep) femoral artery
right internal iliac artery
descending branch of lateral circumflex artery
genicular arteries
right popliteal artery
right superficial femoral artery
right anterior tibilal artery
right posterior tibial artery
right peroneal artery
right dorsalis pedis artery
planter arch

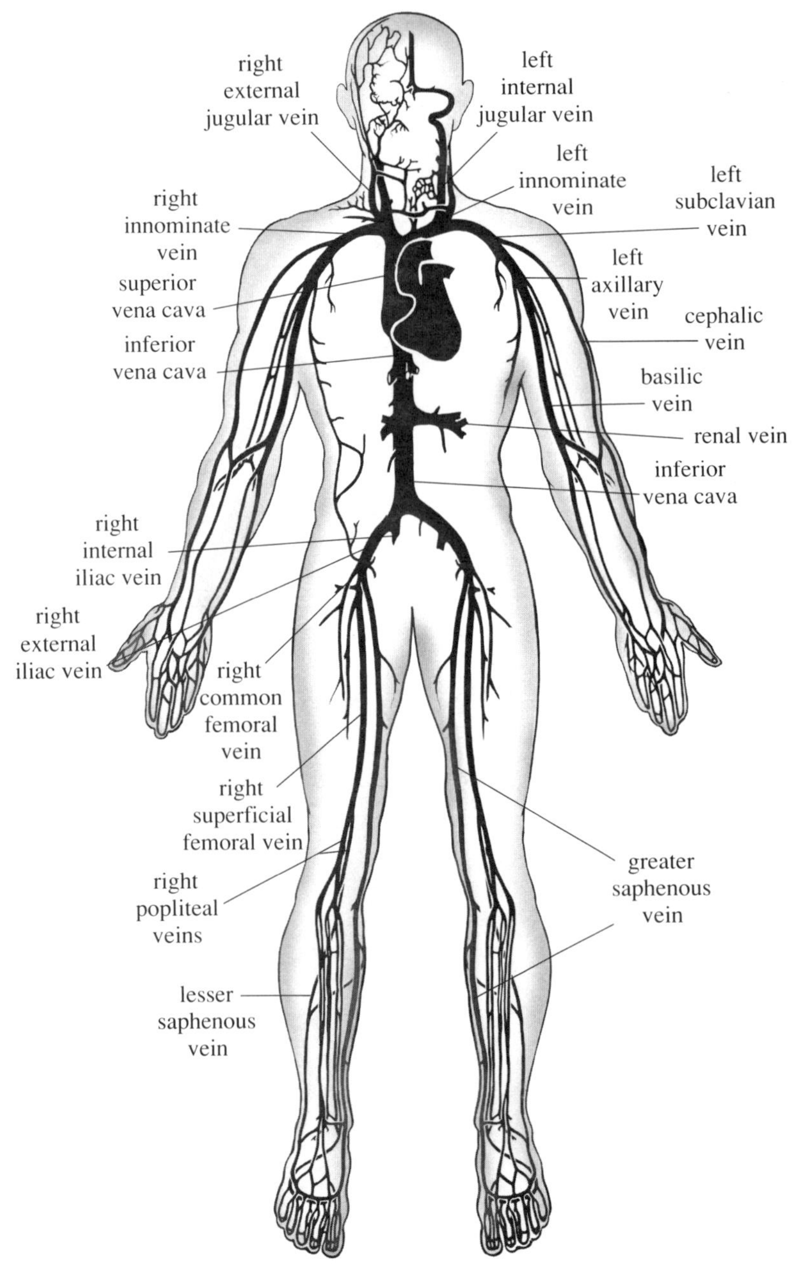

right external jugular vein
left internal jugular vein
left innominate vein
left subclavian vein
right innominate vein
superior vena cava
left axillary vein
inferior vena cava
cephalic vein
basilic vein
renal vein
inferior vena cava
right internal iliac vein
right external iliac vein
right common femoral vein
right superficial femoral vein
greater saphenous vein
right popliteal veins
lesser saphenous vein

Chapter One

Angina

What is angina?

Angina is a medical term used to describe chest discomfort resulting from a momentary lack of blood flow to the heart muscle. The heart is a powerful, muscular pump which requires a constant supply of nutrients and oxygen. This nutrient and oxygen supply is furnished only by the coronary arteries which run on the surface of the heart. Much like the root system of a tree, the coronary arteries send small branches into the substance of the heart muscle, or myocardium, to supply individual muscle fibers with food and oxygen. If the coronary arteries become narrowed due to deposits of cholesterol-laden material, called atherosclerosis, then a region of heart muscle is deprived of needed blood flow (Figure 1-1).

This lack of blood flow is particularly apparent during periods of physical exertion. Angina may then be manifest as a pressure-like or squeezing discomfort located beneath the breastbone. This discomfort may radiate to the arms, neck, shoulders or jaw. The situation is much like the discomfort produced by wrapping a rubber band tightly around the tip of one's finger. When the finger is exercised by flexing backward and forward, the aching discomfort due to lack of blood flow becomes more severe. If the finger is

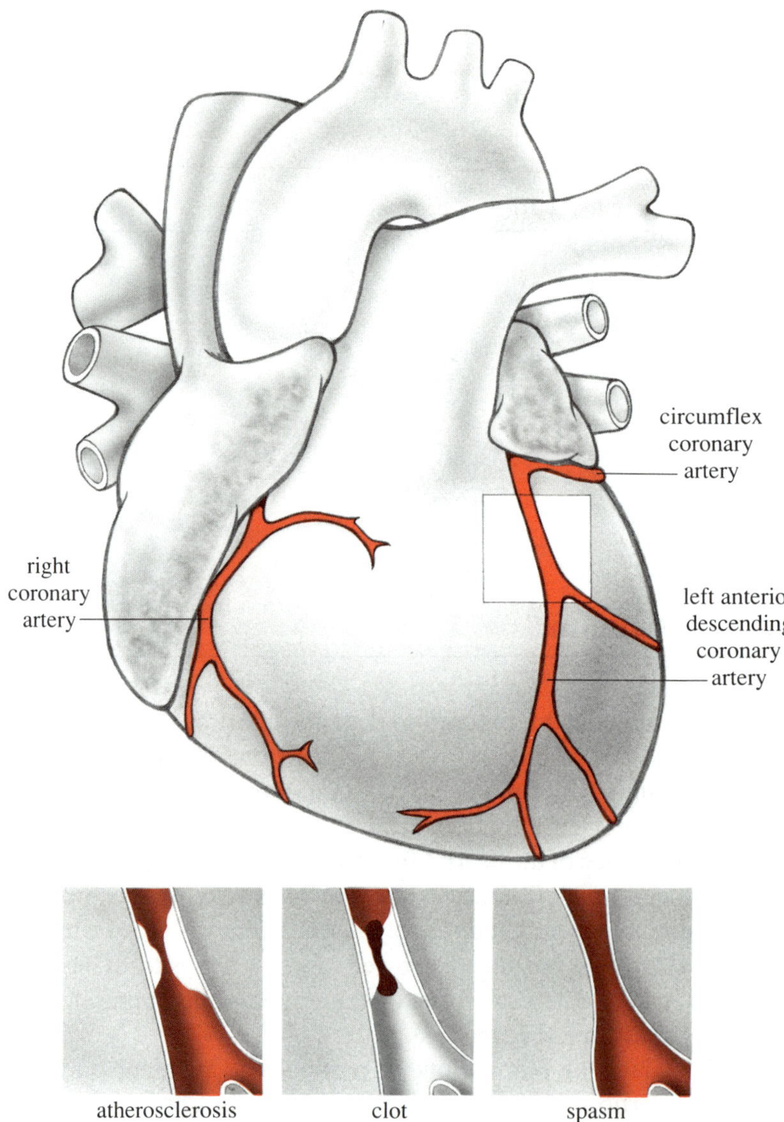

Coronary artery atherosclerosis and spasm generally produce intermittent chest pain, or *angina*, but do not result in permanent heart muscle damage. However, complete coronary occlusion by blood clot causes irreversible heart muscle damage, or *heart attack*.

rested or the constricting rubber band removed, the discomfort lessens and eventually disappears.

Angina is, therefore, a temporary imbalance between the demand of the heart muscle for oxygen and nutrients and the ability of the coronary arteries to supply those nutrients (Figure 1-2). Angina episodes do not result in damage to the heart muscle since the imbalance of blood flow is a reversible event and can be relieved by rest or use of medication such as nitroglycerin. In contrast, heart attack, or *myocardial infarction* (MI), occurs when permanent and irreversible damage to the heart muscle is brought about by a complete blockage of coronary blood flow. This happens when an area of coronary atherosclerosis suddenly ulcerates or "blisters" producing a clot overlying the atherosclerotic deposit. The clot then completely plugs the already narrowed coronary channel and causes a complete cessation of coronary blood flow. If the blood flow is not restored within a matter of hours, the region of heart muscle supplied by the blocked artery is irreversibly damaged and eventually replaced by scar tissue.

Heart attack symptoms are usually much more severe than angina and persist despite rest or use of nitroglycerin (Table 1-1). A heart attack is often described as if "someone is sitting on the chest" and may be associated with nausea, vomiting, profuse sweating, generalized sense of weakness, and a sense of impending doom. Most patients who have angina learn to recognize its characteristic features and can readily distinguish between an episode of angina and a heart attack. If symptoms suggestive of heart attack occur, you should seek immediate medical attention. Time is of the essence in treatment of heart attack since under some circumstances new medications can be given to dissolve the offending coronary artery clot and restore blood flow. This new therapy, called *thrombolysis*, derives its name from *thrombus*, which means blood clot, and *lysis*, which means to dissolve. Thrombolysis offers the hope of stopping a heart attack thereby limiting the extent and severity of heart muscle damage.

One of the key elements for success in thrombolytic therapy is *prompt treatment*. In the event of a heart attack, it is essential to avoid delay and seek immediate care at the nearest hospital. Unfortunately, many heart attack victims fail to recognize or deny the early symptoms and may try a variety of home remedies before reporting to the emergency room. It would be far better to discover your chest pain is a "false alarm" than to reduce the benefits of early heart attack treatment by unnecessary delay.

Figure 1-2   ANGINA– AN IMBALANCE BETWEEN CORONARY ARTERY BLOOD SUPPLY AND HEART MUSCLE DEMAND

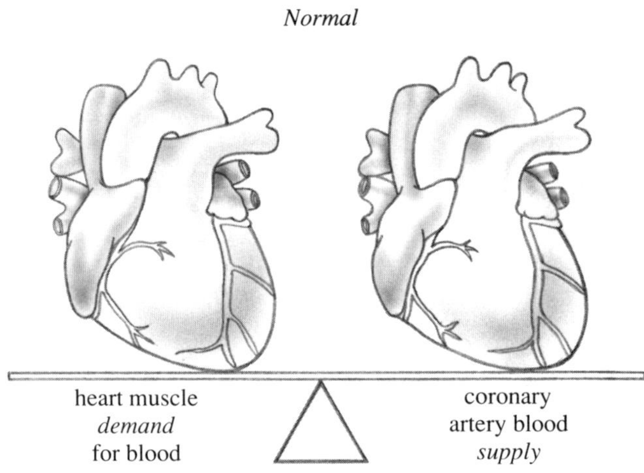

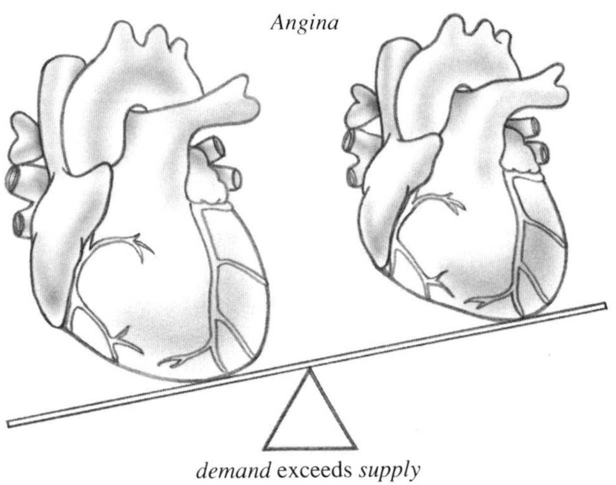

Table 1-1 WARNING SIGNS OF HEART ATTACK

❑ Pressure or squeezing discomfort in the middle of the chest lasting for several minutes or longer.

❑ Spreading of the chest pain into the neck, jaw, shoulder or arms.

❑ Sweating, nausea, vomiting, shortness of breath or fainting

❑ If some of these warning signs appear, *don't delay;* **seek immediate medical attention.**

How is angina diagnosed?

Your doctor often gains clues as to whether angina is present based upon a careful history and physical examination. Since angina is a temporary imbalance of blood flow to the heart muscle, *effort angina*, is often provoked during periods of physical or emotional stress. Heavy meals may also trigger some episodes of angina. Occasionally patients experience what is termed *mixed angina*. Patients with mixed angina experience chest discomfort not only with effort but also experience angina at times of rest. This happens when spasm of the muscular coronary artery occurs in the same region as an atherosclerotic plaque (Figure 1-1). The constriction produced by spasm and plaque narrows the blood vessel sufficiently to impede blood flow at rest and produce anginal symptoms.

Oftentimes patients with mixed angina develop chest discomfort at a particular time of day such as during morning or evening hours when coronary spasm may be more prominent. Like the exertional episodes of chest discomfort, anginal pains due to coronary spasm are often relieved by the use of nitroglycerin. Rarely, patients may experience angina solely due to spasm of a coronary artery without any associated underlying atherosclerotic narrowing. This uncommon form of angina is termed *Prinzmetal's angina* after the physician who first described its occurrence. Prinzmetal's angina often produces chest discomfort unrelated to physical activity.

The character of your chest pain, its timing, location and aggravating influences provides your doctor with important diagnostic clues. However, certain diagnostic tests are also extremely helpful in determining if the symptoms are due to coronary artery disease.

The *electrocardiogram*, called an EKG, measures the electrical activity of the heart as it contracts. If an area of heart muscle has been previously damaged by heart attack, the resulting scar is "electrically silent". This may produce characteristic changes on the electrocardiogram providing evidence of past heart attack.

An electrocardiogram at rest, however, provides only limited information about the coronary circulation. More often it is necessary to record a series of electrocardiograms while the heart performs increasing levels of work-load during exercise. This test, termed an *exercise electrocardiogram* or *stress test*, may reveal telltale signs of coronary artery obstruction (Figure 1-3). However, it is important to understand that the exercise electrocardiogram does not directly measure coronary blood flow but measures only the electrical activity of the heart.

Electrical activity of the heart is in fact very sensitive to changes in coronary artery blood flow, and thus, the stress test is an indirect measure of coronary flow. As such, there are certain limitations of exercise electrocardiography. First, a stress test generally will not detect obstructions to coronary blood flow until the artery is at least 50% reduced in cross-sectional diameter. Second, despite the presence of advanced coronary artery disease, some patients may simply demonstrate no EKG abnormalities during testing. Such a test result is termed a "false negative" study. Third, some patients may demonstrate an abnormal exercise electrocardiogram tracing yet ultimately be found to have no evidence of coronary artery obstruction. This test response, termed a "false positive", is more likely to occur in young and middle-aged females.

Despite the statistical limitations caused by false positive and false negative results, the exercise electrocardiogram remains one of the most useful tools at your cardiologist's disposal. In the vast majority of patients, it serves as a very effective method to screen for the presence of coronary artery disease. It should be remembered, however, that the test is an indirect method for assessing coronary artery blood flow and as such has inherent limitations. It is best to think of the test not as a full-proof method of diagnosis but rather a means by which your cardiologist can estimate the probability that coronary

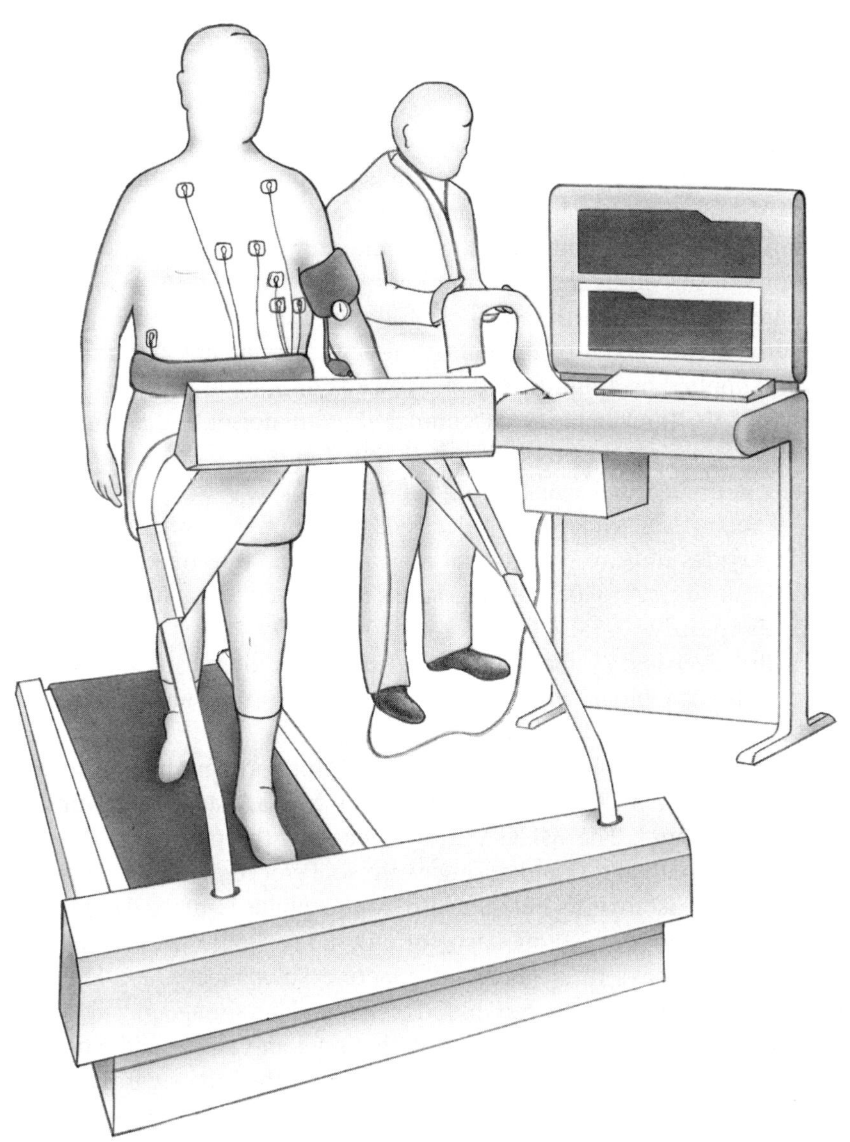

artery blockage is the underlying cause of your chest discomfort. If the test is inconclusive, or if it indicates the presence of potentially significant coronary artery disease, your cardiologist may well recommend additional testing such as cardiac catheterization or nuclear cardiac studies.

One of the most common nuclear cardiac studies performed is the *thallium exercise electrocardiogram* (Figure 1-4). This test is conducted in much the same way as the exercise electrocardiogram. The patient walks on a treadmill belt which gradually increases in both speed and incline. The EKG is continuously monitored for any abnormality suggestive of impaired coronary blood flow. At peak effort, an injection is performed through an intravenous line (I.V.) placed in the hand or arm prior to the test. This injection contains a small amount of radioactive isotope, thallium 201 chloride, which is then promptly absorbed by the heart muscle in direct proportion to blood flow in each area of the heart. Immediately following exercise, thallium activity is measured in each of these segments using a nuclear camera. A segment of heart muscle supplied by a significantly narrowed coronary artery will demonstrate decreased thallium activity as compared with normal adjacent segments. Routine follow-up images performed four hours post exercise help locate regions of myocardial scar due to past heart attack.

As compared with exercise electrocardiography, exercise thallium testing often provides improved statistical accuracy. Thallium treadmill testing is a very useful adjunct to the standard stress test, especially in patients who may have false positive or false negative exercise EKG changes. It is also a helpful test if the electrical system of the heart has been altered by the presence of "bundle branch block". A normal test provides reassuring evidence that coronary circulation is in fact normal.

Another form of nuclear cardiac testing for coronary heart disease is the *rest and exercise MUGA study* (Figure 1-5). MUGA stands for "multi-gated angiocardiogram". The MUGA study measures the pumping action of the heart muscle both at rest and during exercise. Prior to the test, a trace amount of a radioactive isotope, technetium 99 pyrophosphate, is injected intravenously. As with thallium, this isotope lasts for only a few hours within the body and then rapidly decays to an inert and inactive substance. Once injected, the isotope attaches itself to red blood cells and an image of the pumping chambers, or ventricles, is obtained with a nuclear camera and a computer.

Of particular interest is performance of the main cardiac pumping chamber, the left ventricle. Since this chamber performs five times the work load of any other heart chamber, abnormalities in coronary artery blood flow are most often reflected by changes in left ventricular pumping action. This pumping response can be measured by the MUGA study both at rest and during

The thallium exercise study reveals regions of poor coronary blood flow caused by atherosclerotic coronary blockage.

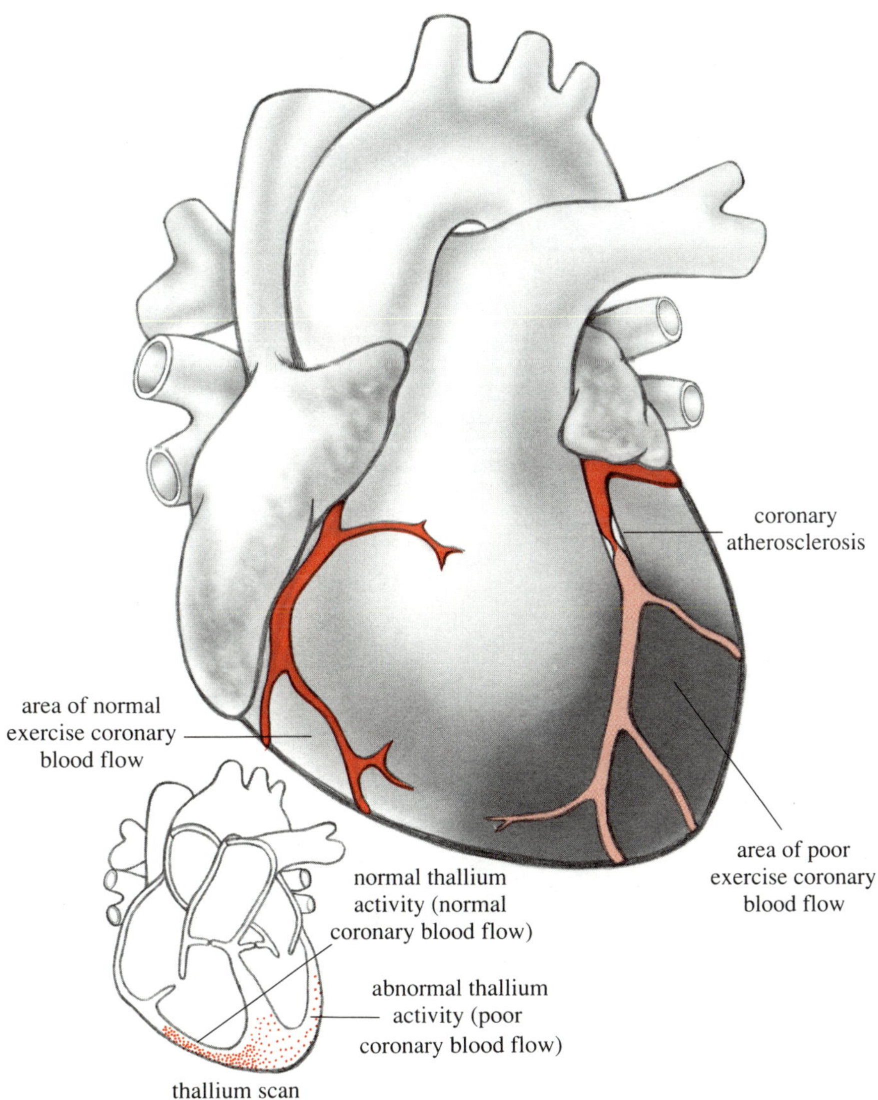

The fraction of blood expelled from the left ventricle during systolic contraction, called the *ejection fraction*, is an important measure of over-all heart muscle function.   At rest, the left

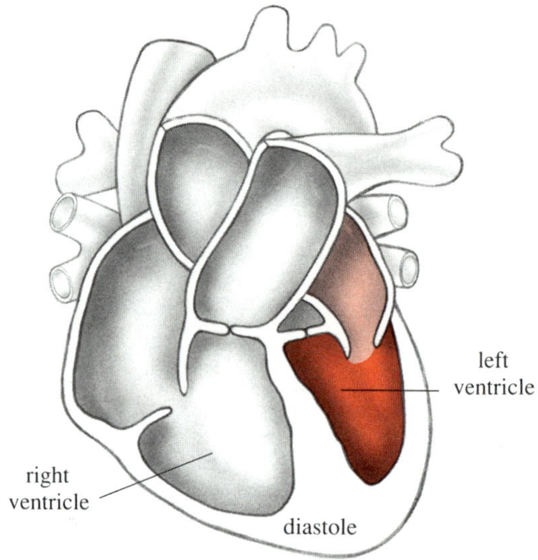

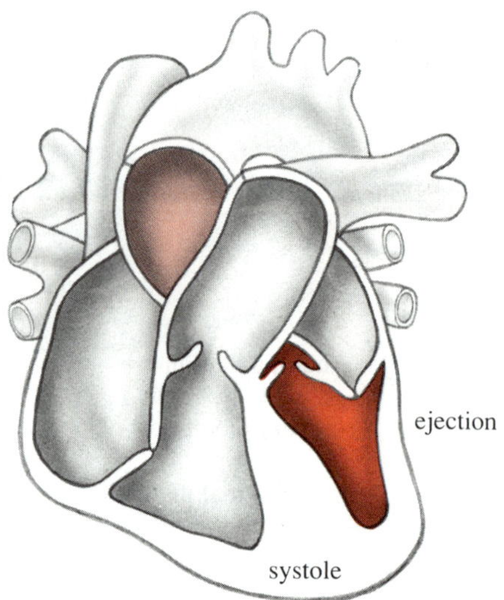

ventricular ejection fraction is 55% or greater. Resting values less than this may indicate abnormal heart muscle function. The ejection fraction increases above resting values with exercise - failure of exercise ejection fraction to increase may indicate poor coronary artery blood flow.

exercise. During the exercise study, the patient typically pedals a bicycle attached to a special imaging table while the exercise electrocardiogram is continuously monitored. Performance of the left ventricle is measured at peak effort and compared with similar images obtained with the heart at rest.

Just as your heart pounds harder within the chest as you dash up a flight of stairs or when you become emotionally excited, the left ventricle pumps more forcibly during normal exercise. If, however, nutrient blood flow to the heart muscle is blocked by coronary artery disease, the pumping action of the heart will not rise in normal fashion during exercise and areas of heart muscle may in fact become sluggish relative to adjacent normal heart muscle segments.

Ventricular performance is measured by computing the fraction of blood expelled from the heart with each beat termed the *ejection fraction*. The ejection fraction normally increases with exercise. A failure of the ejection fraction to increase with exercise as measured by the MUGA study or a fall from normal values, is a sensitive indicator of coronary artery disease. MUGA testing is typically done in a specialized laboratory and may take several hours to complete. There is no significant discomfort during either the thallium or MUGA tests, and the risks of study are minimal. *However, as with any x-ray study, **it is important you inform the technician or cardiologist if there is any chance you are pregnant.***

What is cardiac catheterization?

If your history or noninvasive studies such as exercise treadmill testing or nuclear cardiac scan raises the suspicion of significant coronary artery disease, additional testing such as cardiac catheterization may be advised. During cardiac catheterization, a series of small flexible plastic tubes, termed catheters, are carefully directed through the circulatory system to the coronary arteries (Figure 1-6). X-ray dye is then injected directly into the coronary arteries and 35 mm. motion pictures, called coronary arteriograms, are obtained. Other catheters are advanced into the cardiac chambers where pressure is measured and additional x-ray dye (ventriculogram) injected to examine the pumping action of the left ventricle. These pictures and pressure measurements provide precise information as to the extent and severity of coronary artery blockage as well as vital data regarding heart muscle and valve function. This information can be of fundamental importance in planning your future therapy and in determining your overall prognosis.

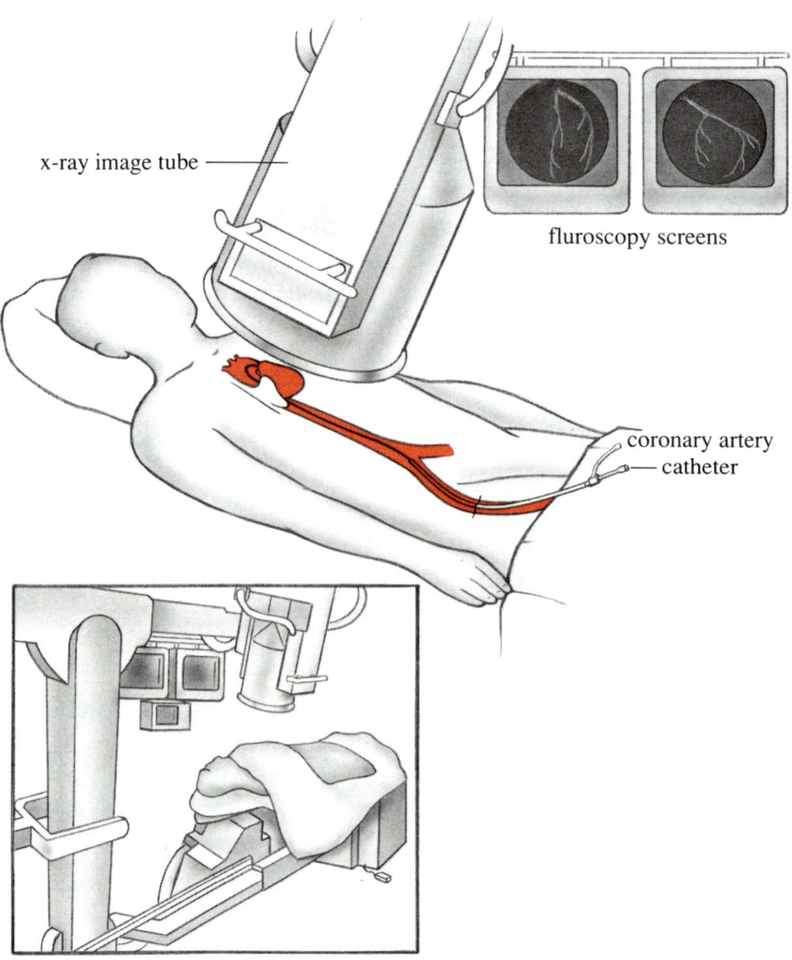

x-ray image tube
fluroscopy screens
coronary artery
catheter

Cardiac catheterization findings may indicate a need to modify your medical therapy or indicate a need to consider other means of treatment such as coronary balloon dilation (coronary angioplasty) or coronary bypass graft surgery.

Cardiac catheterization is performed in a specially-equipped hospital laboratory (*cath lab*) specifically designed to obtain high resolution images of the coronary artery circulation. You are awake during the procedure and experience only minimal discomfort as the blood vessel near the groin crease (femoral artery) or elbow region of the arm (brachial artery) is anesthetized with local xylocaine. Since there are no nerve fiber endings on the interior of blood vessels, there is no discomfort or sensation as the catheters are subsequently advanced into the arteries and moved into position. A mild sensation of warmth is felt as the x-ray dye is injected into the main pumping chamber of the heart, but this warm flushing sensation quickly disappears after approximately thirty seconds.

Upon conclusion of the procedure, all catheters are removed and pressure applied at the needle puncture site if the femoral artery approach is used or the arm incision site is closed with suture if the brachial artery approach is used. Should the femoral artery be used, you will be instructed to lie still in bed with the catheterization leg immobile for a number of hours during which time a sandbag may be placed over the groin artery to prevent leakage of blood (Table 1-2).

Although complications can occur during cardiac catheterization, the overall complication rate is less than 1% in most circumstances. This includes the risks of injury to a blood vessel or nerve, infection, bleeding, disturbance of cardiac rhythm, heart attack, stroke, death, or allergic reaction to x-ray dye or medication. Some bruising at the catheterization site is a normal occurrence and is not a cause for alarm. This bruising represents a small volume of blood which seeps out around the catheter while it is in the artery during the catheterization procedure. The discoloration gradually subsides over several weeks and then disappears. A small pea-sized scar nodule may remain at the catheterization site for many years and is also a normal occurrence. If, however, at any time after the procedure you experience pain or swelling at the catheterization site, notice leg numbness or weakness, or any other bothersome symptoms, you should report them immediately to your attending nurse or cardiologist. ***It is important to tell your cardiologist before the catheterization if you are allergic to x-ray dye, iodine compounds, or iodine-rich seafoods such as shrimp, lobster, clams or oysters.***

The information provided by your cardiac catheterization is often crucial not only in further clarifying your diagnosis but also in selecting the most

Table 1-2	**PATIENT INSTRUCTIONS FOLLOWING HEART CATHETERIZATION**

❑ Report any

    ❑ chest discomfort

    ❑ pain, swelling or bleeding at catheterization site

    ❑ numbness, discomfort or swelling of the leg or arm used for catheterization

    ❑ unusual or new symptoms

❑ Follow your post-catheterization activity instructions closely. Don't move the leg or arm used for catheterization until specifically instructed to do so.

❑ Stay at bedrest until instructed otherwise. During this time, keep your head against the pillow and avoid straining or coughing. Use the bed pan or urinal as needed.

❑ Drink plenty of fluids to help remove the x-ray dye (contrast) from your body.

❑ Avoid heavy exertion of the arm or leg used for catheterization for 3 to 5 days. Report any new or persistent catheterization site swelling, numbness, discomfort, redness, pain, fever, or unusual symptoms.

appropriate treatment for your particular condition. Therefore, the benefits of cardiac catheterization far exceed the small risks involved.

In summary, angina is diagnosed by a careful history and physical examination in conjunction with a variety of specialized diagnostic tests. These tests are often used in combination with one another since the information they provide is often additive and complimentary to each other.

How is angina treated?

Although there is no true cure for coronary artery disease, its symptoms and natural progression can often be relieved and changed by a variety of new treatment modalities. Combined with adjustments in lifestyle, these treatments allow most patients with angina to continue an active life and maintain gainful employment.

Since angina is an imbalance between the demand of the heart muscle for oxygen-rich blood and the ability of narrowed coronary arteries to supply those nutrients, treatments directed to correct this imbalance of supply and demand are often very effective.

What medications are used for treatment of angina?

A variety of medications are used to treat angina (Table 1-3). They principally work by reducing the demand of the heart muscle for nutrient supply. This is accomplished by increasing the mechanical and chemical efficiency of the heart muscle pump. In this manner, the heart is able to perform its function despite impairment of coronary blood flow. This is analogous to improving the mechanical efficiency of an automobile engine by adjusting the carburetor mixture setting or adding an overdrive gear to the transmission, thus extracting more miles to each gallon of gas.

Nitroglycerin is the oldest form of medication used for the treatment of angina. In general terms, nitroglycerin works by reducing internal left ventricular filling pressures and by dilating the coronary arteries. Nitroglycerin may be taken as needed in tablet or spray form beneath the tongue during angina or in anticipation of physical or emotional stress likely to provoke an anginal attack.

Generic Names	*Common Brand Names*
Nitrates	
nitroglycerin	Nitrostat®, Nitro-Bid®, Nitrodisc®
	Transderm-Nitro®, Nitro-Dur®
	Nitropaste®, Nitrolingual Spray®,
	Nitroguard®
isosorbide dinitrate	Isordil®, Sorbitrate®
Calcium Channel Blockers	
diltiazem	Cardizem®
nifedipine	Procardia®
verapamil	Calan®, Isoptin®
nicardipine	Cardene®
Beta Blockers	
atenolol	Tenormin®
labetalol	Trandate®, Normadyne®
metoprolol	Lopressor®
nadolol	Corgard®
pindolol	Visken®
propanolol	Inderal®, Inderal-LA®
timolol	Blocadren®

Nitroglycerin typically produces a slight burning sensation beneath the tongue and may be associated with a momentary headache in some individuals. Nitroglycerin tablets can taken safely during an anginal episode every two to three minutes. However, if pain relief is not obtained after approximately three nitroglycerin tablets or if angina-like discomfort persists beyond fifteen minutes, it is best to seek immediate medical attention. Such an episode may not be angina but represent early symptoms of a heart attack.

Because nitroglycerin works by lowering blood pressure, it may also produce a momentary sense of light-headedness. Be prepared to sit down and place your head between your knees if this occurs, or better yet, to lie down if circumstances permit. Most patients tolerate nitroglycerin exceptionally well and receive prompt anginal relief with its use.

Nitroglycerin products may also be taken periodically during the day in sustained release oral tablets such as isosorbide dinitrate, or be delivered continuously to the circulation by use of topical nitroglycerin patches or nitroglycerin paste. These forms of nitroglycerin are most useful in patients who have frequent episodes of angina and in whom the use of sublingual nitroglycerin tablets may be inconvenient or ineffective in preventing angina. Nitroglycerin tolerance may develop with use of nitroglycerin patches, paste or sustained release tablets. That is, the response of the heart to a given nitroglycerin dosage may lessen as a result of continuous exposure to nitroglycerin. This is much like the phenomenon of tolerance to a bothersome odor which develops after prolonged exposure to the smell. After a while you become unaware the offensive odor is present. In the same fashion, your heart and circulation can become tolerant to the beneficial effects of nitroglycerin. Your doctor may, therefore, periodically review and change your dosage if evidence of nitroglycerin tolerance is present.

Because nitroglycerin is a volatile substance and may evaporate from the matrix of the sublingual tablets, it is best to replace your supply of nitroglycerin tablets every three months. This will assure availability of a potent and effective dose when you need it. Alternatively, nitroglycerin spray, available in a small canister, provides long-lasting nitroglycerin potency with a long-lasting shelf life.

Another group of anti-anginal medications is the *beta blockers*. Beta blockers work by reducing the oxygen demands of the heart muscle by slowing heart rate, reducing blood pressure, and by reducing the contracting force of heart muscle fibers. By reducing these factors, beta blockers serve to decrease the energy demands upon the heart muscle and thereby reduce the need for oxygen-rich coronary blood flow. Asthmatic patients or those with emphysema may experience increased difficulty with breathing on beta blockers and may not be able to use these medications. Brittle diabetes or poor circulation to legs may also be aggravated by beta blockers. Occasionally patients complain of sleep disturbance or fatigue on beta blockers and this may necessitate the use of an alternate medication.

More recently a group of compounds termed *calcium channel blocking agents* have entered the scene for the treatment of angina. These medications have a variety of effects on coronary blood flow and heart muscle function combining many of the activities of both nitrates and beta blocking agents. Like nitrates, the calcium channel blocking agents are effective in relaxing the muscle envelope around the coronary artery, thus reducing the occurrence of spasm in patients with either mixed angina or Prinzmetal's angina. They also reduce the demand of the heart muscle for blood flow, thus helping to stabilize the imbalance of supply and demand in patients with effort angina. Side effects may include constipation, headache, swelling of the feet and rarely fluid congestion within the lungs.

What is coronary bypass surgery?

If medical therapy is ineffective for relief of angina and if it appears as though substantial areas of heart muscle are at risk for future heart attack, your cardiologist may advise coronary bypass graft surgery. Bypass surgery works by directly increasing the *supply* of blood flow to the heart muscle via grafts which detour blood around coronary artery obstructions (Figure 1-7). Coronary bypass surgery is performed by opening the chest cavity through an incision in the mid-line of the breastbone (sternum). Through tubes entering the chest cavity, the circulatory system is connected to an artificial heart-lung pump. Body temperature is then cooled and heart pumping action momentarily ceases while heart and lung function is assumed by the heart-lung bypass pump. Cessation of heart activity allows the surgeon to construct grafts on the surface of the heart.

Segments of saphenous vein are removed from the leg and a small opening made in the coronary artery beyond the area of obstruction. One end of the vein is then sewn onto the coronary artery and the other end is sewn onto a small opening made in the aorta. Blood then enters the vein graft from the aorta and detours around the coronary blockage. Once the grafts are completed, the heart is stimulated to beat once again and the patient is weaned off the bypass pump.

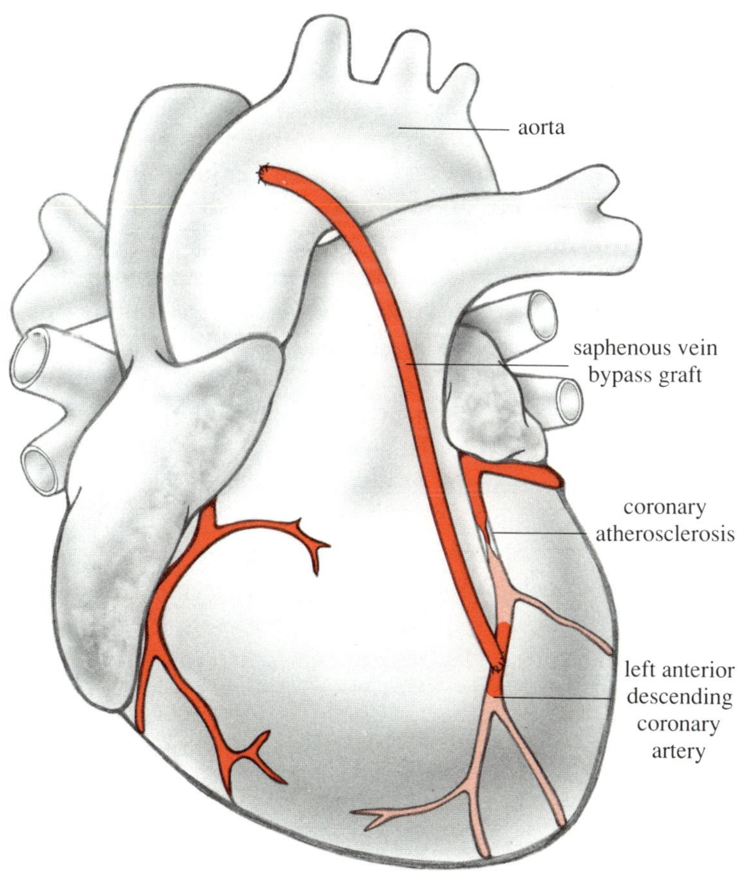

aorta
saphenous vein
bypass graft
coronary
atherosclerosis
left anterior
descending
coronary
artery

In many cases it is also possible to sew an artery from within the chest wall, called the internal mammary artery, onto one or perhaps two coronary arteries to establish what is termed an internal mammary artery bypass graft (Figure 1-8). The specific circumstances of surgery may not always permit the use of an internal mammary artery graft, but when possible, mammary grafting often provides greater graft durability than with saphenous vein grafting.

It is clear that coronary bypass graft surgery can be very effective in relieving angina in patients for whom medical therapy is ineffective. In certain select groups of patients, such as those with left main coronary artery obstruction, those with multiple coronary artery blockages, and those with impaired heart muscle pumping action, coronary bypass surgery has also been shown to improve long-term survival. Vein bypass grafts, however, do generally develop progressive atherosclerosis which may become an important problem approximately ten years following surgery. In addition, it is not possible in some circumstances to effectively construct bypass grafts to diffusely diseased coronary arteries or to coronary vessels which may be inherently small in size. Such grafts are at increased risk for closure with blood clot, since the slow, somewhat stagnant blood flow run-off in these grafts promotes blood clotting and graft closure. Patients with a significantly weakened heart muscle, of advanced age, or who have associated medical illnesses of significant nature such as diabetes, lung or kidney disease, are clearly higher risk surgical candidates.

Therefore, the decision to proceed with coronary bypass graft surgery is based upon a careful analysis of the cardiac catheterization findings, severity of the patient's anginal symptoms, an appraisal of his general medical condition, as well as a careful analysis of his risk for complications of coronary bypass graft surgery. In many patients, the benefits of surgery clearly outweigh the associated risks and offer the patient years of additional life with substantially reduced anginal symptoms.

What is coronary angioplasty?

Beginning in 1977, an innovative technique for the treatment of coronary artery obstructions was pioneered by Dr. Andreas Gruntzig in Zurich, Switzerland. This technique, *p*ercutaneous *t*ransluminal *c*oronary *a*ngioplasty (PTCA), uses a small balloon-tipped catheter to open areas of narrowing within the coronary artery system (Figure 1-9). Using a technique much like

INTERNAL MAMMARY (THORACIC) ARTERY BYPASS SURGERY

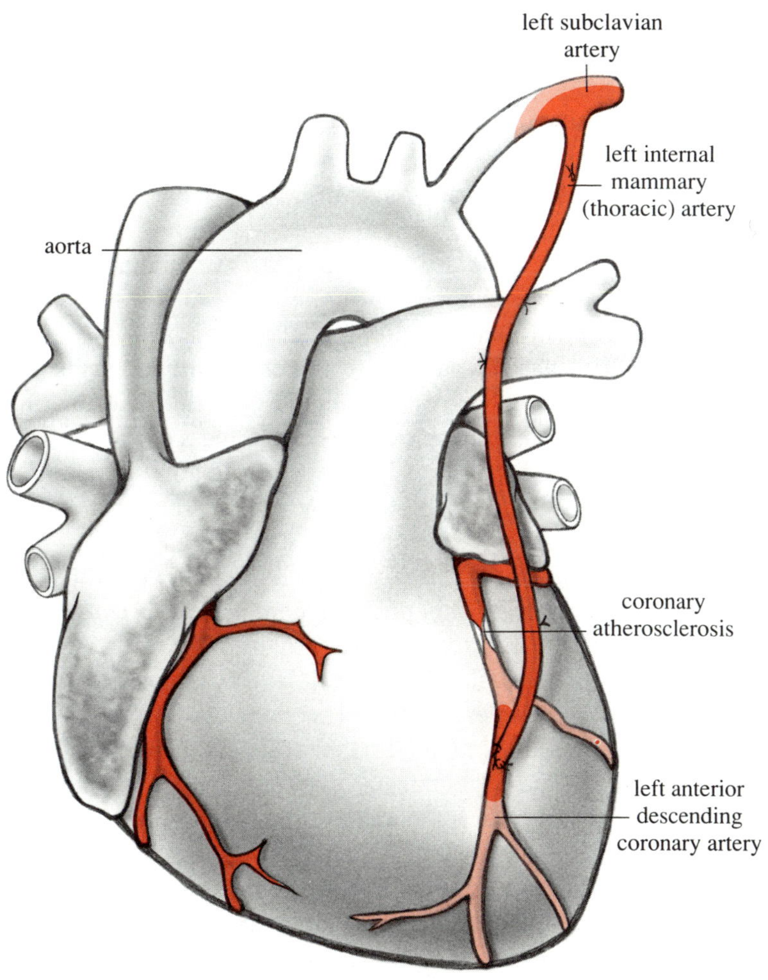

cardiac catheterization and with the patient awake in a mildly sedated condition, a small catheter with a collapsed balloon is carefully advanced over a guide wire into the site of coronary obstruction. Under x-ray guidance, the balloon is then inflated thereby compressing the atherosclerotic material against the wall of the vessel and stretching the elastic envelope of the coronary artery. This is much like compacting freshly fallen snow with one's footprint. The net result is a wider channel for coronary blood flow and relief or reduction in anginal symptoms.

Coronary bypass graft surgery detours blood around coronary blockages and does not cure the underlying atherosclerotic plaque. Similarly, coronary angioplasty is not curative for coronary artery disease but remodels the vessel interior and may result in many years of improved coronary blood flow and reduced anginal symptoms.

Occasionally the coronary artery may fail to open during angioplasty or may suddenly close due to appearance of either a small blood clot or a small tear (dissection) on the interior of the coronary artery. This may result in a need for immediate coronary bypass graft surgery. Cardiac surgical standby is therefore available in advance of angioplasty. Informed consent for both coronary angioplasty and emergency coronary bypass graft surgery is obtained prior to proceeding with balloon dilation in order to allow expeditious surgical treatment if needed. Fortunately, *sudden* closure of a coronary artery during balloon dilation occurs infrequently.

Following hospital discharge, the dilated vessel is carefully observed for any signs of renarrowing. This phenomenon, called *restenosis*, occurs as a natural part of the healing process in perhaps 25% to 30% of all patients following coronary angioplasty (Figure 1-10). Restenosis is *not* caused by a recurrence of the atherosclerotic plaque but rather by the gradual deposition of scar tissue on the interior of the blood vessel at the dilation site. Usually this scar tissue is only tissue-paper thin and does not obstruct coronary blood flow. However, in 25% to 30% of patients this scar tissue formation may be significant and impair blood flow. Just as a skin incision heals in some patients with minimal scarring and in others with a more apparent incisional scar, the coronary artery may heal with variable amounts of scar tissue from patient to patient. If restenosis occurs, it is often feasible to redilate the blood vessel with repeat angioplasty. Restenosis most often appears within the first three to six months following coronary angioplasty. A recurrence of angina greater than six months post angioplasty is usually *not* due to restenosis but rather due to progression of atherosclerotic disease at other locations in the coronary artery system.

Thus, it is important to understand that for some patients coronary

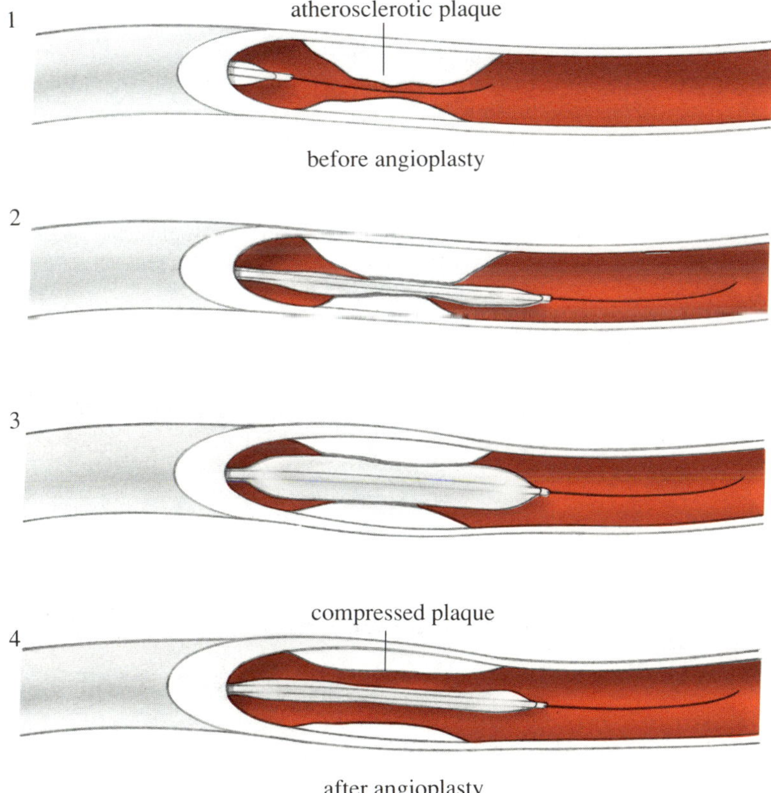

1
atherosclerotic plaque
before angioplasty
2
3
compressed plaque
4
after angioplasty

TREATMENT OF CORONARY RESTENOSIS BY REPEAT BALLOON ANGIOPLASTY

Following balloon angioplasty natural healing processes may in some patients renarrow the vessel. This is usually successfully treated by repeat dilation.

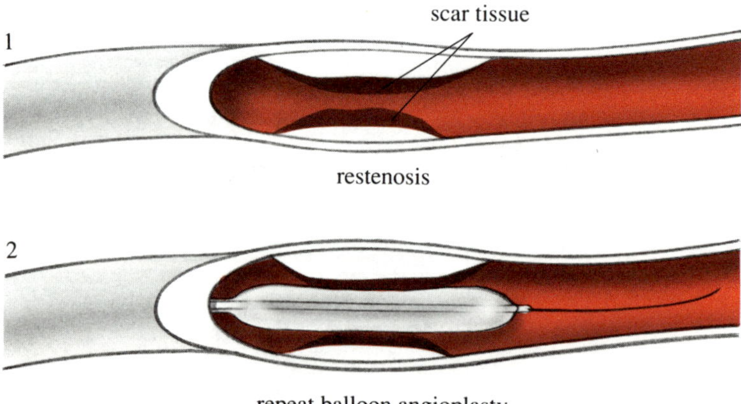

angioplasty may be a two-step procedure: an initial dilation to compact the atherosclerotic plaque and stretch the vessel channel followed at a later date by a follow-up dilation to stretch any scar tissue which may form. When restenosis is a recurring problem for a given patient, coronary bypass graft surgery is often considered as an alternate solution. Extensive scientific research is presently under way to better understand the mechanism of restenosis and hopefully will provide future methods for its prevention.

Is exercise of benefit for treatment of angina?

Exercise is very useful for controlling coronary heart disease risk factors and improves the overall efficiency of the heart and circulatory system. By improving the efficiency of the circulatory system, the supply-demand imbalance of coronary blood flow in angina may be substantially reduced.

A program of physical activity should be undertaken only after conferring with your personal physician. He may suggest an exercise treadmill test in order to formulate an exercise prescription. The exercise prescription outlines the intensity of exercise as well as the type and duration of exercise appropriate for your heart condition.

What are the known risk factors for coronary disease?

Control of risk factors for coronary artery disease is essential in every angina patient. Atherosclerosis can result in progressive narrowing of the coronary arteries and attention to underlying risk factors can retard its progression. High blood pressure, smoking, high blood cholesterol, obesity, and diabetes are risk factors which may be modified or controlled by medical therapy or changes in diet and lifestyle. Some risk factors for coronary artery disease can't be changed such as if you have a family history of early coronary disease under the age of 50, if you are male, or if you are over 40 years of age. Therefore, it is important that every effort be made to modify those risk factors which are under your control.

What is unstable angina?

In many patients, angina has a characteristic pattern and does not change significantly despite the passage of years. However, if angina suddenly increases in frequency and severity, then the term *progressive* or *unstable angina* applies. Recent studies have demonstrated that unstable angina is often associated with disruption of the atherosclerotic plaque and associated clot formation.

Since this is the sequence of events which may lead to complete coronary occlusion and myocardial infarction, unstable or progressive angina demands immediate medical attention.

Therefore, if a change in your usual anginal pattern is noticed, be certain and report promptly to your doctor for further evaluation.

What causes chest pain other than angina?

A large number of structures within the chest cavity can produce pain and discomfort mimicking angina. Unfortunately, disorders of many internal body organs produce rather nondescript discomforts which are very similar even though they may come from entirely different organs.

For example, inflammation of the swallowing tube, or esophagus, behind the heart may produce a sense of burning discomfort in the chest identical to angina. Spasm of the esophagus may also produce angina-like discomfort and surprisingly this spasm is also relieved with nitroglycerin, further confusing the issue. Ulcers within the stomach (peptic or duodenal ulcers) may also produce discomfort which radiates into the chest cavity, mimicking angina.

Often inflammation of the lining membrane around the lung (pleurisy) or lining membrane around the heart (pericarditis) produces sharp, "knife-like", chest discomfort. This pain may confuse itself with angina, but unlike angina, it lasts only a few seconds and is aggravated by deep breathing. Arthritis in the chest wall or inflammation of the ligaments, muscles or tendons of the chest cavity can produce musculoskeletal discomfort similar to angina.

Other times, inflammation of the gallbladder (cholecystitis), liver inflammation (hepatitis), pneumonia, an expanding aortic aneurysm or an aortic dissection can produce symptoms similar to that of heart attack.

Therefore, the diagnosis of coronary artery disease and angina pectoris is oftentimes a difficult diagnostic challenge for your physician. You can help in this effort by making note of the character of your pain, its location, its aggravating factors, as well as those factors which produce relief of the discomfort. This information, coupled with your physical examination and diagnostic tests, will provide your physician with important insights into your condition.

What is the role of aspirin in the treatment of heart disease?

Since heart attacks result when a blood clot obstructs a coronary artery at the site of atherosclerotic narrowing, treatment designed to reduce the likelihood of blood clot formation is of clear importance.

The first step in blood clot formation is the clumping together of small circulating packets in the bloodstream called platelets. Aspirin has been discovered to inhibit the clumping of platelets, thus reducing the likelihood of clot formation. Initial studies investigating the use of aspirin in heart disease demonstrated a reduction in the risk of *second* heart attack in patients taking aspirin following an initial heart attack.

Recently however, the Physician's Health Study from Harvard Medical School, as reported in the *New England Journal of Medicine* on January 28, 1988, demonstrated that aspirin was effective in reducing the risk of an initial heart attack.

This study involved 22,071 male physicians. One-half of this group was administered aspirin 5 grains (325 mg.) every other day, and the remaining group of physicians was administered placebo (a tablet containing no medication).

The study demonstrated a 47% reduction in the occurrence of heart attack in a five year follow-up period among those physicians taking the aspirin dosage.

Although this information is exciting news, it is somewhat tempered by the risk of stroke reported in the study. There was a 15% increase in overall risk of stroke in the study which was not statistically significant. However, those strokes caused by moderate, severe, or fatal bleeding within the brain did occur more frequently among the aspirin-treated group. This subgroup of strokes was statistically important although it is important to note it involved a very small number of patients (10 in the aspirin group and 2 in the placebo group).

Should aspirin be taken by all persons?

Before considering lifelong aspirin therapy, it is important to understand the concerns raised by the Physician's Health Study. Since high blood pressure increases the risk of stroke, aspirin therapy should be considered very carefully in patients with *uncontrolled* high blood pressure. Furthermore, it is important to understand that aspirin does not reduce the underlying atherosclerosis but simply reduces the risk of clot formation within an atherosclerotic vessel. Therefore, principle attention should be directed towards reducing the underlying risks for atherosclerosis such as cigarette smoking, hypertension, and high blood cholesterol.

The American Heart Association recommends the following practical guidelines related to the use of aspirin:

1. Aspirin should be taken on an every-other-day basis only after consultation with your physician. Certain illnesses such as kidney and liver disease, peptic ulcer, or intestinal bleeding may be aggravated by aspirin therapy. Bleeding disorders or use of anticoagulant therapy would contraindicate the use of aspirin. Your physician will be able to advise you as to the relative risks of chronic aspirin therapy.
2. The principle risk factors for heart disease and stroke should be determined and a plan of action to control these risks be undertaken before beginning a lifelong aspirin therapy program.
3. It is important to understand the possible risks of aspirin therapy including possible bleeding complications. Aspirin should be discontinued before many forms of surgery since aspirin may affect the blood clotting process for as much as ten days after stopping the drug.

Heart disease remains a major cause of death in the United States, and therefore the news regarding aspirin and its role in the reduction of heart attack death rate is certainly good news. However, aspirin does not prevent underlying atherosclerosis and does have certain side effects which may outweigh the potential benefits in a given patient. Therefore, before undertaking life-long aspirin therapy, be certain and check with your physician to determine if the benefits outweigh the potential risks.

Chapter Two

Heart Attack

What is a heart attack?

In medical terms, heart attack describes the process which occurs when an area of heart muscle is completely deprived of blood supply. This occurs when a coronary artery on the surface of the heart becomes completely blocked depriving a segment of heart muscle of nutrient and oxygen supply. If this obstruction is not promptly reversed, an area of heart muscle (*myocardium*), undergoes a process of deterioration termed *infarction* and is eventually replaced by scar tissue. Thus, the medical term for heart attack is *myocardial infarction* (MI for short).

In recent years, it has been established that most heart attacks occur due to the sudden occlusion of a coronary artery by blood clot. This typically occurs overlying an area of atherosclerotic build-up within the coronary. The inciting event is usually rupture of an atherosclerotic plaque which results in the formation of a blood clot. New therapeutic strategies for the treatment of heart attack employ clot dissolving medication to restore coronary blood flow. Today, with the availability of such treatment techniques, prompt treatment and evaluation of heart attack is therefore of utmost importance.

New therapy for heart attacks.

Prior to the advent of clot dissolving medications, therapy for heart attack was limited to providing bed rest and supportive treatment for complications of heart attack. Today, clot dissolving medications, called thrombolytic agents, offer a new opportunity to actually limit the extent of heart muscle damage, thus improving heart function and saving lives (Figure 2-1).

The fluid state of the blood is naturally maintained in a delicate equilibrium between the competing processes of blood clot formation and blood clot dissolution. Thrombolytic drugs act by stimulating the clot dissolving properties of blood. The two most common thrombolytic drugs used for heart attack treatment in the United States today are streptokinase and tissue plasminogen activator (tpA). Both of these medications can be given during heart attack by intravenous infusion. Although streptokinase and tissue plasminogen activator have revolutionized the treatment of myocardial infarction, *it is important to understand that these drugs **cannot** be used for treatment of heart attacks in **all** patients.*

The use of thrombolytic therapy entails certain risks, and on occasion the risk of bleeding complication or other difficulties may exceed the anticipated benefits of treatment. In general terms, patients who are the best candidates for treatment with thrombolytic agents fall into two groups. First are patients who present for treatment within the first 4-6 hours of heart attack. During this period of time, reopening of the vessel may save substantial areas of heart muscle from permanent damage. Because the loss of heart muscle is an on-going and continuous process beginning at the moment of coronary occlusion, greatest benefit of thrombolytic therapy occurs when it is given within the first few hours following onset of heart attack (Figure 2-2). The second group of patients who benefit substantially from thrombolytic therapy are those with large heart attacks. Restoration of coronary blood flow in these patients can reduce the likelihood of extensive heart muscle damage.

Our understanding of thrombolytic therapy and identification of those patients most likely to benefit from treatment is undergoing a process of rapid change and evolution. One of the most difficult tasks facing both patient and physician is determining whether the benefits of thrombolytic therapy exceed the anticipated risks. Clearly each case must be approached on its individual merits and an expeditious treatment decision made based upon a careful analysis of the available medical facts. Because thrombolytic therapy promotes dissolution of blood clots, there is always a risk of internal bleeding including the potential for brain hemorrhage and stroke. In addition to the risk of internal

HEART ATTACK: TREATMENT WITH THROMBOLYTIC AGENTS

Heart attack is caused by a blood clot which forms over an atherosclerotic coronary plaque.

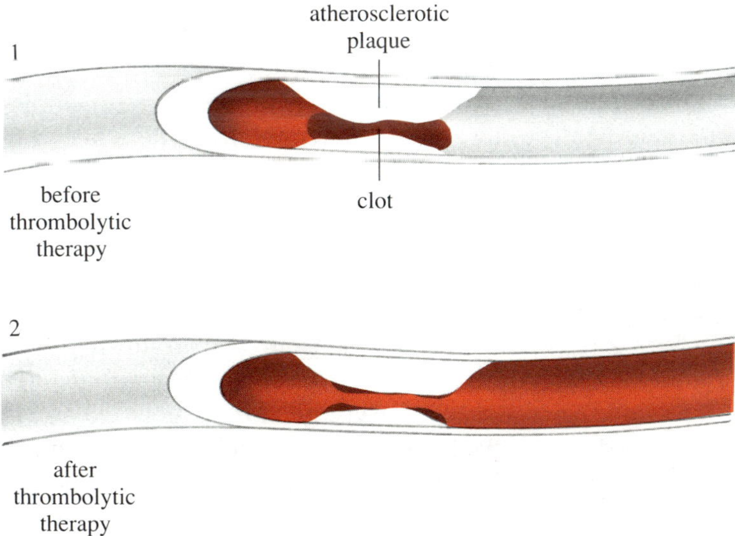

Thrombolytic agents may dissolve most of the blood clot, but a severe plaque and residual narrowing may persist.

bleeding complications, thrombolytic therapy may also be associated with certain serious cardiac rhythm disturbances which are usually momentary in nature.

In appropriately selected patients, the risks of these complications are low, especially when one considers the substantial benefits of thrombolytic therapy. The recently completed GISSI (*Gruppo Italiano Studio Streptochinase Infarto Miocardio*) study demonstrated that thrombolytic therapy within the first hour of heart attack may reduce the risk of death by as much as 47% (Figure 2-3). Because of its potential for substantial reduction in heart attack mortality and its proven effectiveness in limiting the extent and severity of heart muscle damage during heart attack, thrombolytic therapy has become one of the most powerful tools in the cardiologist's armamentarium.

Obstructed coronary arteries can be opened in approximately 60% to 80% of cases treated with thrombolytic therapy. Although the offending blood clot is partially dissolved and forward coronary blood flow restored, a significant residual blockage composed of underlying atherosclerotic plaque and blood clot remnants may remain. Sometimes this residual blockage is severe and persistent, posing a risk for recurrent heart attack or severe angina. Cardiac catheterization may be performed at some point following thrombolytic therapy to determine if additional measures such as balloon dilation (coronary angioplasty) are needed to open a wider channel for coronary blood flow. For other patients, cardiac catheterization may reveal a need for coronary bypass surgery or a modification of medical therapy.

The timing and need for cardiac catheterization following thrombolytic therapy is an individualized and flexible decision. Data reported in the 1988 TIMI - II b study (*Thrombolysis In Myocardial Infarction*) indicate that some patients can be safely observed on medical therapy after thrombolysis and then treated with coronary angioplasty or coronary bypass surgery at a later date should problems develop. In many patients thrombolytic therapy is a temporary measure designed to stop a heart attack which must be combined at a later time with further treatment to restore coronary blood flow to more normal levels.

The clot dissolving action of thrombolytic agents are short- lived, lasting only several hours. Clot dissolving drugs are therefore combined with anticoagulants such as heparin, aspirin or dipyridamole (Persantine®) to prevent rapid reaccumulation of blood clot over the ulcerated atherosclerotic plaque. Other medications such as nitroglycerin compounds and calcium channel blocking agents may be used to reduce coronary artery spasm in the heart attack-related vessel.

Emergency coronary bypass graft surgery and emergency coronary angioplasty have also been used as effective treatment strategies for the

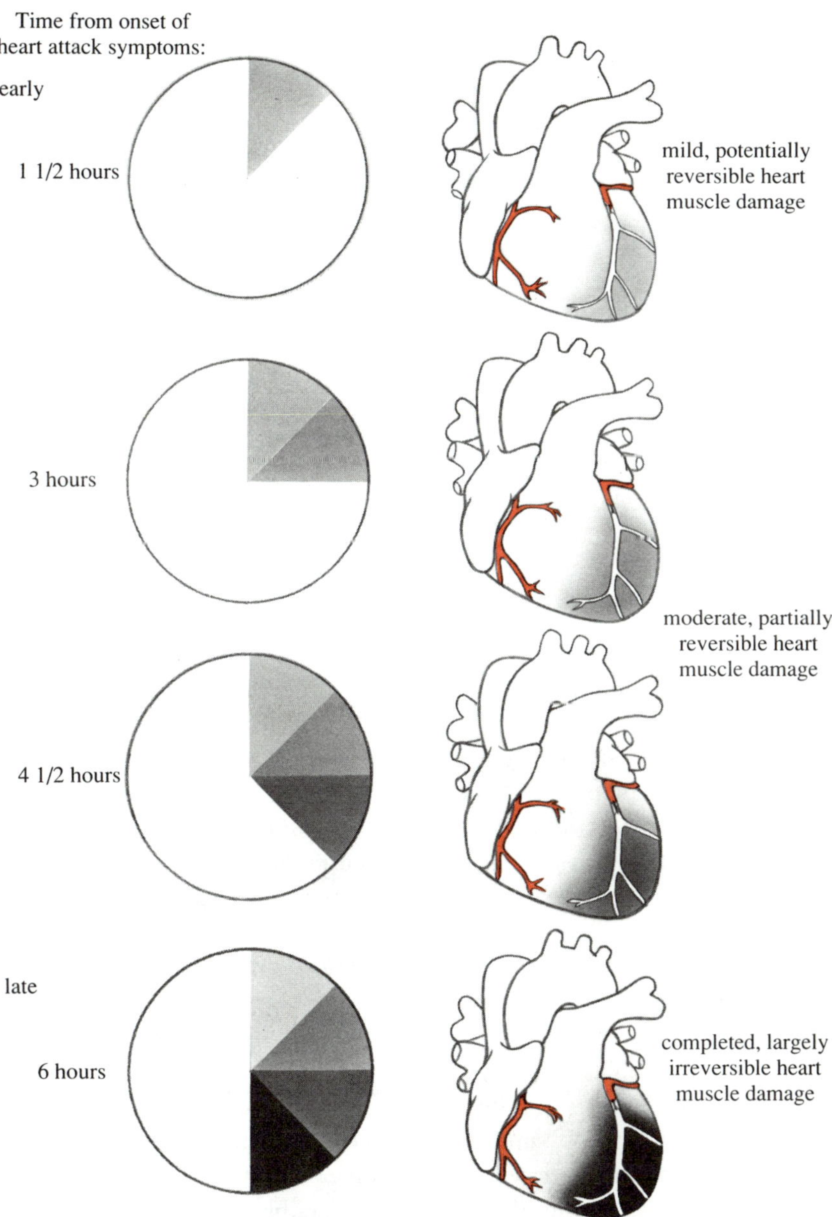

Heart muscle damage begins at the moment of coronary occlusion. If the coronary artery remains closed, heart muscle damage is usually complete and irreversible within 4-6 hours.

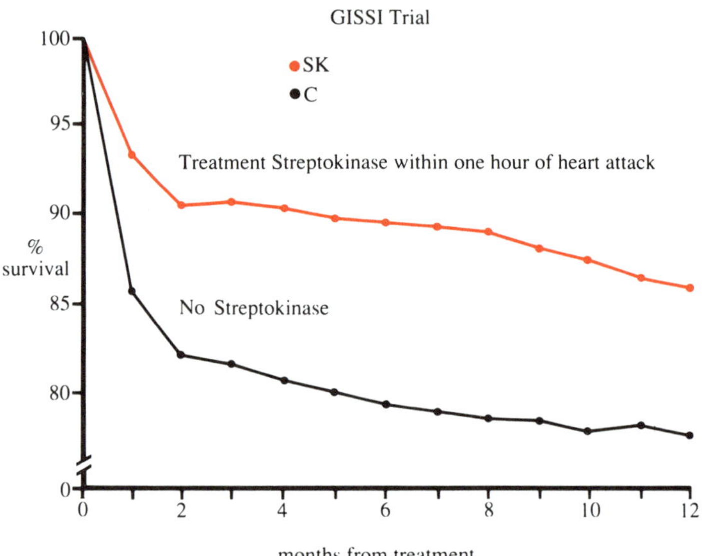

treatment of heart attack; however, the logistics and increased risks of performing these complex procedures during the early hours of a heart attack generally restricts their use to special circumstances.

If your doctor advises the use of thrombolytic treatment for heart attack, he will carefully explain the relative risks and benefits of this treatment as they may relate to your specific condition. It is important to tell your doctor as much as possible about your past medical history especially any history of previous stroke, bleeding ulcers, recent surgery, or prior therapy with streptokinase (Table 2-1). Although there are established *absolute* contraindications to thrombolytic therapy, usually contraindications, if they exist, are *relative* contraindications and must be carefully weighed against the potential benefits of prompt coronary thrombolysis. If following a discussion of the risks and benefits of thrombolytic therapy both you and your physician decide to proceed with such treatment, he will ask you to sign an informed consent document indicating your understanding of the treatment and its potential risks, benefits and alternatives. Circumstances permitting, your doctor will attempt to involve your family as much as possible in discussions regarding thrombolytic therapy and may ask your nearest of kin to cosign the consent form with you.

        **THINGS TO TELL YOUR DOCTOR BEFORE
                      RECIEVING THROMBOLYTIC THERAPY**

Tell your doctor if you have any of the conditions listed below:

❏   Recent bleeding or know bleeding disorder

❏   History of stroke

❏   History of ulcers

❏   Recent surgery (especially in the past two months)

❏   History of brain tumor, brain artery aneurysm or other brain circulation
     problems

❏   Recent injuries (especially to the spinal column or head)

❏   Heart valve disease (especially mitral stenosis)

❏   Severe uncontrolled high blood pressure

❏   Diabetic or other retinal eye disease

❏   Pregnancy

❏   Current or recent use of anticoagulants (blood thinners)

❏   Any condition in which bleeding would be anticipated

❏   Prior history of having received streptokinase therapy

Devices and medications for heart attack treatment.

Thrombolytic therapy clearly represents one of the most important breakthroughs in the treatment of myocardial infarction. This breakthrough treatment has also been complimented by advancements in supportive drug treatment for heart attack and new devices for monitoring and assisting the failing circulation during heart attack.

Myocardial infarction may be associated with a drop in blood pressure due to a deterioration in the pumping action of the heart muscle. *Vasopressor agents* such as *dopamine* and *dobutamine* may be used to stimulate cardiac contraction and maintain blood pressure. A newer agent, *amrinone* (Inocor®) has also proven to be an extremely useful medication to support the failing heart muscle.

When medications for supporting blood pressure fail or if increasingly severe anginal episodes follow a heart attack, your cardiologist may advise insertion of an intra-aortic balloon pump (Figure 2-4). The intra-aortic balloon pump is a small balloon envelope connected to a hollow tube. It is inserted by first administering local anesthesia near the groin artery and then, either using a small incision or a needle puncture, inserting the balloon into the artery and advancing it to a position in the aorta near the heart. During the relaxation phase (diastole) of each heart contraction, the balloon inflates, displacing blood along the aorta thereby augmenting the pumping action of the heart muscle. As with all foreign objects in the circulation, there is a risk of blood clot formation around the balloon catheter with possible dislodgement (embolization) of these clots to other vital areas of the circulatory system. The shaft size of present day aortic balloon pump catheters has been reduced significantly in size, yet the shaft may nonetheless impair blood flow to the leg used for balloon insertion. These complications may require discontinuance of the balloon pump or construction of a bypass graft channel to the leg to improve blood flow.

Your cardiologist may also advise insertion of a Swan-Ganz® catheter into the heart and lungs (Figure 2-4). Under local anesthesia, this small balloon tipped catheter is introduced via a neck vein (internal jugular vein) or groin vein (common femoral vein). The catheter provides precise diagnostic measurement of blood pressure within the lungs and of heart filling pressure.

The electrical system of the heart may be damaged during heart attack resulting in a variety of heart rhythm disturbances. Excessive slowing in the heart rate (bradycardia) may occur and increase the risk for sudden stoppage of all cardiac activity (asystole). In these circumstances, a temporary pacemaker

DEVICES FOR MONITORING AND SUPPORT OF THE HEART ATTACK PATIENT

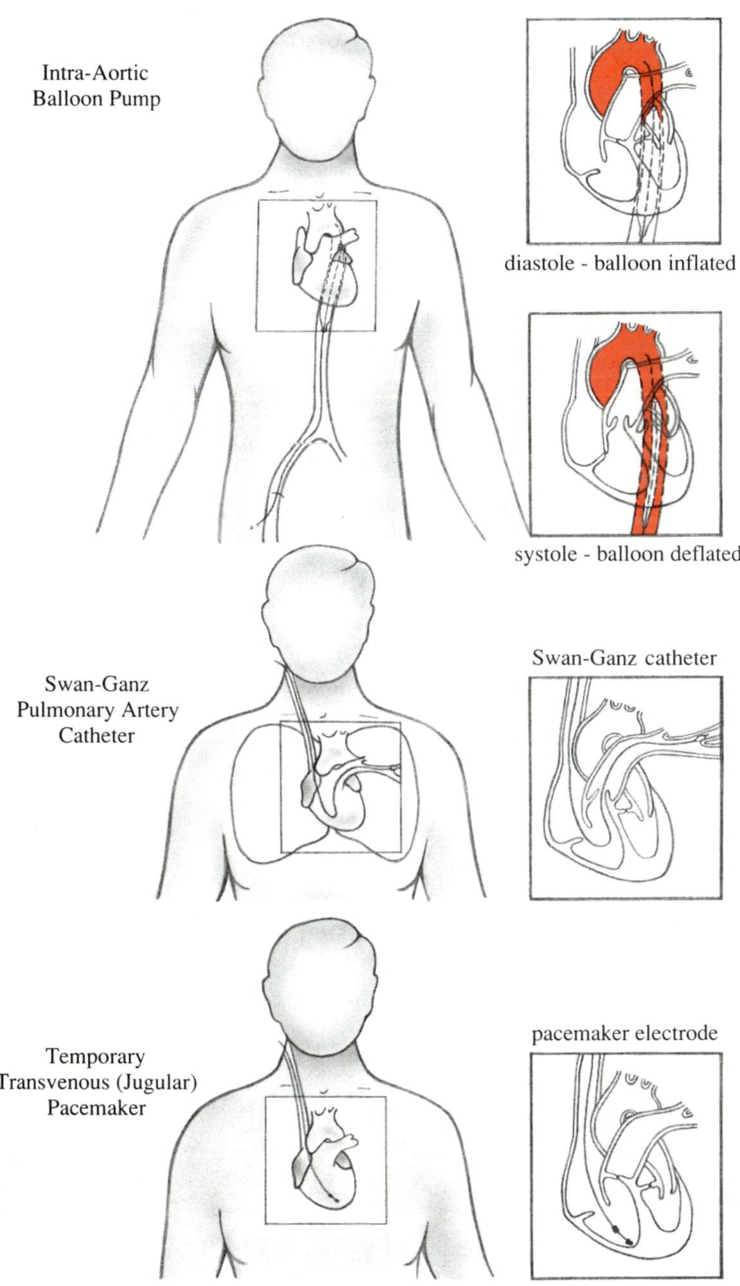

is needed (Figure 2-4). It is inserted in a fashion essentially identical to placement of the Swan-Ganz® catheter and is connected to a small battery pack and timing circuit located at the bedside. Once the pacemaker is no longer needed, it is simply removed and a bandage placed over the entry site. Another effective means for pacing the heart rhythm during heart attack involves placement of large electrode pads on the chest wall such that small currents of electricity can be passed through the heart thereby maintaining a steady rhythm. This technique, called *transcutaneous pacing*, is usually used as a precautionary measure in those patients at increased risk for slow heart rhythm or when pacing is needed quickly or for only a short period of time.

While hospitalized in the coronary care unit, the heart rhythm is continuously monitored and should a heart rhythm abnormality be noted, anti-arrhythmic therapy may be prescribed. The purpose of these medications is to reduce the likelihood of more serious forms of heart rhythm disturbance. A variety of medications are commonly employed and again must be individualized based upon the type and severity of heart rhythm disturbance observed. *Lidocaine* and *procainamide* are two of the most commonly used intravenous agents for treatment of arrhythmia during myocardial infarction.

Figure 2-5   **CARDIAC ENZYME LEVELS FOLLOWING HEART ATTACK**

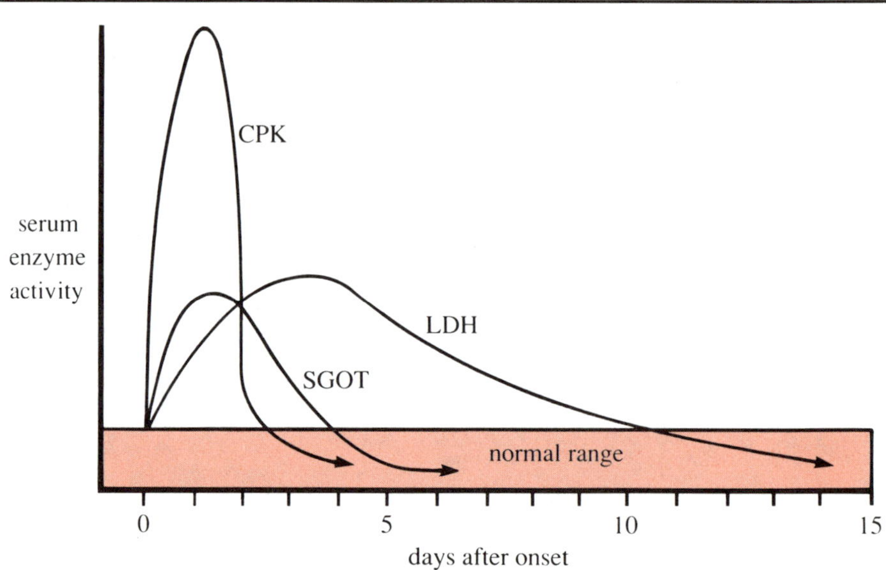

How is a heart attack diagnosed?

Just as there have been significant advancements in the treatment of heart attacks, the ability to detect heart muscle injury has also been substantially improved over the last decade. However, the electrocardiogram remains a cornerstone of heart attack diagnosis. The EKG is a measure of the electrical activity of the heart and sudden injury to the heart muscle due to an occluded coronary artery will change the EKG pattern within moments following occlusion. The EKG is therefore a very early indicator of heart attack and is used extensively for heart attack diagnosis.

The heart muscle, like all body tissues, contains large amounts of chemicals called *enzymes* which are responsible for controlling a number of important biochemical reactions within each heart muscle cell. If the muscle cell is permanently damaged and undergoes cell death, the envelope that surrounds the cell, termed the cell membrane, becomes leaky and releases some of these enzymes into the bloodstream.

Cardiac enzymes such as CPK, SGOT, and LDH can be detected in the blood by standard laboratory tests and elevated cardiac enzyme levels confirm the presence of heart attack. The release of each cardiac enzyme occurs in a slow progressive manner with an initial rise in CPK followed by a later rise in SGOT and LDH (Figure 2-5). Because of the delay required for cardiac enzymes to appear in the bloodstream, a decision for or against use of thrombolytic therapy is usually based upon symptoms and EKG findings. The subsequent rise in cardiac enzymes confirms the EKG diagnosis and provides clues as to whether the coronary artery has been reopened (reperfused) by thrombolytic therapy. If the vessel has been reperfused, there will often be a brisk and large increase in the blood level of cardiac enzymes. As noted earlier, additional testing such as treadmill examination or cardiac catheterization is usually required to determine if the offending blood clot has been adequately dissolved.

Chapter Three

Cardiovascular Disease Risk Factors

What are the known risk factors for cardiovascular disease?

A number of factors have been identified by years of careful scientific study as significantly increasing a person's risk of developing atherosclerosis. Since atherosclerosis is a major cause of death and disability in the United States and leads to conditions such as heart attacks, stroke, kidney disease and arterial insufficiency of the legs, it is important to understand what these risk factors are and how they may be modified to reduce the risk of cardiovascular disease (Figure 3-1).

The following factors significantly increase the risk of atherosclerosis:

1. Smoking
2. High blood pressure (hypertension)
3. Elevated blood cholesterol (hypercholesterolemia)
4. Diabetes
5. Strong family history of cardiovascular disease
6. Male sex
7. Obesity
8. Physical inactivity

The role of a stressful lifestyle as an independent predictor of risk for cardiovascular disease continues to be strongly debated.However, in many circumstances, such a stressful lifestyle may worsen or contribute to the above known risk factors.

The present scientific evidence suggests the following practical approach toward management of cardiovascular risk factors: (1) Maintain a body weight as close to ideal as possible (Table 3-1); (2) Do not smoke; (3) Engage in regular exercise. Before starting a new exercise program, be certain it is medically safe to do so; (4) If you have certain medical conditions such as high blood pressure or diabetes, obtain and follow appropriate therapy; (5) Follow a heart healthy diet.

Figure 3-1   EFFECT OF MULTIPLE POSITIVE CARDIAC RISK FACTORS

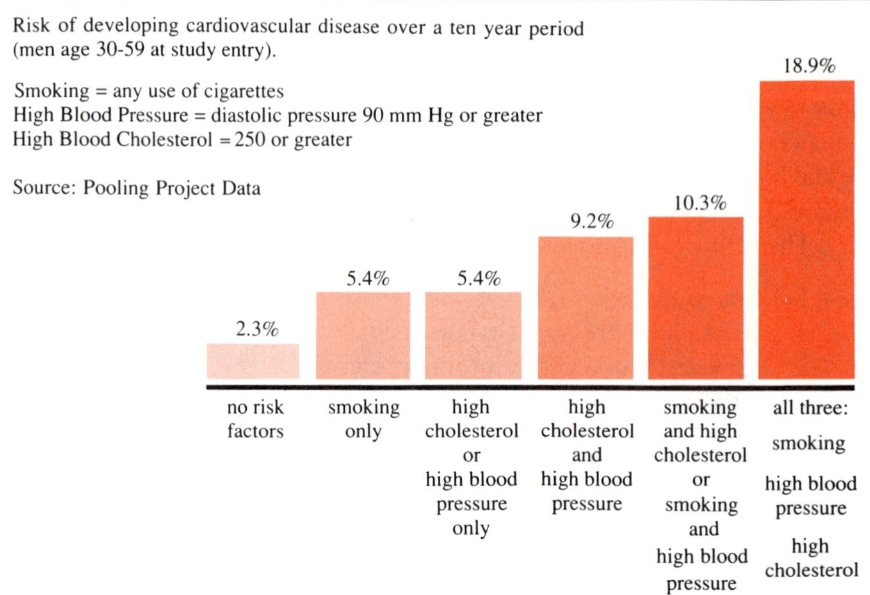

Height Without Shoes	*Weight Without Clothes*	
	Men (pounds)	Women (pounds)
4' 10"	—	92-121
4' 11"	—	95-124
5' 0"	—	98-127
5' 1"	105-134	101-130
5' 2"	108-137	104-134
5' 3"	111-141	107-138
5' 4"	114-145	110-142
5' 5"	117-149	114-146
5' 6"	121-154	118-150
5' 7"	125-159	122-154
5' 8"	129-163	126-159
5' 9"	133-167	130-164
5' 10"	137-172	134-169
5' 11"	141-177	—
6' 0"	145-182	—
6' 1"	149-187	—
6' 2"	153-192	—
6' 3"	157-197	—

Note: For women 18-25 years, subtract one pound for each year under 25.
Source: Adapted from the 1959 Metropolitan Desirable Weight Table.

The fat content of your diet should constitute no more than 30% of total calorie intake. The saturated fat intake should be less than 10% of total calories, and polyunsaturated fat intake approximately 10% of total calories. Cholesterol intake should be limited to less than 300 mg. per day. In the sections to follow we will explore some of these concepts in more detail.

What is cholesterol? What is triglyceride?

Blood cholesterol and triglyceride are important components in the formation of atherosclerosis, a fatty build-up of material within the walls of arteries which results in obstruction to blood flow and can lead to heart attack, stroke and other circulatory disorders. The role of cholesterol in the formation of atherosclerosis is now well established by a variety of scientific observations. There is less certainty about the role of triglyceride in the origin of atherosclerotic disease. Cholesterol and triglyceride are referred to as *lipids* which is the scientific term that describes fat-like substances in the blood. Much of the cholesterol in your blood comes from the liver which produces approximately 1,000 mg. of cholesterol each day. Lipids also enter the body via the foods we eat. Because they are oily-like substances and do not mix with the water-like nature of blood, they must be carried through the blood vessels by special proteins called *lipoproteins*.

The most important lipoproteins in the regulation of atherosclerosis are the low density lipoproteins (LDL for short) and the high density lipoproteins (HDL for short).

An imbalance of the amount of LDL and HDL lipoproteins can accelerate the process of atherosclerosis. LDL *promotes* the deposition of cholesterol on the artery walls. HDL, by contrast, helps to *remove* cholesterol from artery walls and return it to the liver for further chemical digestion (Table 3-2). Elevations of total blood cholesterol and LDL levels significantly increase the risk of atherosclerosis. Depressed levels of HDL similarly increase atherosclerotic risk while high HDL levels offer a protective effect against atherosclerosis.

❏ To remember the action of Low Density Lipoprotein (LDL), think of it as "*L*ousy" lipoprotein, or "bad" cholesterol.

❏ To remember the action of High Density Lipoprotein (HDL), think of it as "*H*ealthy" lipoprotein, or "good" cholesterol.

Blood cholesterol levels can be modified in two ways. First, by altering the amount of cholesterol and fatty foods in our diet, and secondly, if needed, by the use of certain medications which alter the manufacture and breakdown of cholesterol.

Cholesterol directly enters the diet from foods of animal origin such as meats, poultry, some seafoods and dairy products (Table 3-3). Egg yolks and organ meats such as kidney and liver are very high in cholesterol content. Foods of plant origin such as fruits, vegetables, grains, cereals, nuts and seeds contain little or no cholesterol.

Saturated fats have an important role in regulating total blood cholesterol and therefore should be restricted to less than 10% of total daily calories. Saturated fats raise the level of cholesterol in the blood and can usually be identified as those fats that harden at room temperature. They are found in abundant quantities in animal products and some vegetable products. Saturated animal fats are principally found in beef, veal, lamb, pork and ham. They also are contained in dairy products such as butter, cream, whole milk and in cheeses made from cream and whole milk. These foods are also important sources of cholesterol and should be avoided for this reason as well.

Food labels list ingredients in order of weight with the ingredient of greatest amount listed first.

Avoid sources of saturated fat and cholesterol from the following list:

- ❑ Fat (animal, bacon, or beef)
- ❑ Chicken Fat
- ❑ Butter or Cocoa Butter
- ❑ Coconut or Coconut Oil
- ❑ Egg & Egg-Yolk Solids
- ❑ Whole-Milk Solids
- ❑ Hardened Fat or Oil
- ❑ Hydrogenated Vegetable Oil
- ❑ Lard
- ❑ Palm & Palm Kernel Oil
- ❑ Vegetable Oil or Vegetable Shortening (may be coconut or palm oils)

Saturated fats are also found in many solid "hydrogenated" vegetable shortenings. These are fats and oils which have been changed from their natural liquid form by chemical means termed "hydrogenation" to become more solid as in margarines and shortenings. Examples of vegetable oils which contain high quantities of saturated fat are coconut oil, cocoa butter, palm oil and palm kernel oil. Although these are often labeled as "cholesterol free", their high content of saturated fat will clearly raise blood cholesterol levels. These oils are often found in commercial bakery products, candies, fried foods, and nondairy milk and cream substitutes.

By contrast, *polyunsaturated fats* actually help lower the level of blood cholesterol by helping rid the body of newly formed cholesterol. These fats are obtained from vegetable oils such as safflower, sunflower, corn, soybean and cotton seed oils. They are usually liquid at room temperature.

The American Heart Association recommends the following guidelines to control the amount and kind of fat you eat:

1. Limit your intake of meat, seafood and poultry to no more than 5-7 oz. per day.
2. Use chicken or turkey (without skin) or fish in most of your main meals.
3. Choose lean cuts of meat, trim off all the fat you see, and throw away the fat that cooks out of the meat.
4. Substitute meatless or "low meat main dishes" for regular entrees.
5. Use no more than a total of 5-8 teaspoons of fat and oils per day for cooking, baking and salads.
6. Use low-fat dairy products.
7. Increase use of fruits, grains and cereals.

Table 3-4   **FOODS HIGH IN SOLUBLE FIBER**
                 (Pectins, Gums)

Pectins	*Gums*
Apples	Oatmeal
Cabbage	Rolled oats
Carrots	Kidney beans
Cauliflower	Lima beans
Citrus fruit	Red beans
Dried peas	White beans
Green pears	Pinto beans
Potatoes	Black beans
Squash	Garbanzo beans
Strawberries	Guar gum

Table 3-5 CHOLESTEROL & SATURATED FAT GUIDE

	Good	*Limit*	*Avoid*
Meat, Poultry Fish, Shellfish	*Lean cuts* of red meat with all visible fat trimmed		"Prime" grade fatty cuts of meat (spare ribs, corned beef, brisket)
Dairy Products	Skim & 1% milk Low-fat buttermilk Low-fat evaporated milk Low-fat yogurt Low-fat cottage cheese, farmer & pot cheese (less than 2-6 gm fat/oz.)	2% milk Plain yogurt Ricotta, part-skim Part-skim hard cheeses "Light" cream cheese & "light" sour cream	Whole milk Condensed milk Cream products Nondairy creamer Hard cheeses Sour cream Cream cheese
Eggs	Egg whites Egg substitutes (cholesterol-free)		Egg yolks
Fats & Oils	Unsaturated vegetable oils (corn, safflower, peanut, olive, soybean, sesame) Soft & liquid margarines	Nuts & Seeds Avocados and olives	Hard margarine and Coconut & palm oils
Bread, Pasta, Beans	Breads Rice Peas & Beans Low-fat crackers Pasta: Spaghetti & macaroni	Commercial biscuits, waffles, cornbreads	Danish pastry, croissants, doughnuts sweet rolls Granola with coconut Snack crackers Egg noodles & egg pastas
Fruits & Vegetables	Frozen, dried or canned fruits		Vegetables in butter or cream sauce

	Good	*Limit*	*Avoid*
Sweets &	Low-fat sherbet	Ice milk	Store-bought pastries
Snacks	& low-fat yogurt	Homemade cookies	cakes & cookies
	Plain popcorn	& cobblers	
	Low-fat cakes	Eggnog	Buttered popcorn
	& cookies		
	Carbonated beverages		
	Tea, coffee		Milk shakes,
	Angel food cake		ice cream

Adapted from National Cholesterol Education Program, National Heart, Lung & Blood Institute, National Institute of Health.

To further control the amount of cholesterol-rich foods in the diet, use no more than three eggs a week including those used in cooking. Limit the use of shrimp, lobster, sardines and organ meats. Recent information indicates that shellfish may include chemicals termed *sterols* which interfere with cholesterol absorption. Thus, one may include bivalves like oysters, clams, and other mollusks in moderation in the diet. Total cholesterol and LDL cholesterol levels are also decreased by some fibers (pectins and gums). Sources of beneficial fiber include oat bran, green beans, other legumes, apples and citrus fruits (Table 3-4).

These rules and concepts may seem complex at first, however, when one understands the basic principles of avoiding foods high in cholesterol or high in saturated fat, it is much easier to plan a practical daily menu (Table 3-5).

Who needs treatment for high blood cholesterol?

A precise definition of what constitutes high blood cholesterol is difficult to establish and should be determined for each patient (Table 3-6). For example, a young patient with known coronary artery disease and high blood pressure would be approached with a more aggressive plan of treatment for hypercholesterolemia than a patient who is in the seventh decade of life and has none of the other known cardiac risk factors. Similarly, if a patient has a depressed HDL level in the presence of other active risk factors such as known coronary heart disease or a strongly positive family history of heart attack, this might warrant specific treatment.

In 1984, an important study called the Coronary Primary Prevention Trial (CPPT) involving 4,000 men with elevated blood cholesterol levels demonstrated that men who lowered their cholesterol levels with diet and drugs had fewer heart attacks and less heart disease in a seven year follow-up. The study provides strong evidence of cardiac risk reduction for a specific population, that is middle-aged men with high blood cholesterol levels treated with diet and medication. However, many researchers believe this study indicates that reducing blood cholesterol levels in other individuals regardless

Table 3-6 CHOLESTEROL RISK LEVELS

Blood Cholesterol Level	Recommendation
Desirable: Below 200	Recheck cholesterol level within 5 years. Monitor your daily intake of saturated fat and cholesterol.
Borderline High: 200-239	Restrict total fats, saturated fats and cholesterol in diet. Recheck cholesterol annually.
Borderline High with Risk Factors*: 200-239	See your doctor to determine your LDL level. Maintain LDL level less than 130. May need medication in addition to dietary measures.
High: 240 and above	Same as borderline high with risk factors.

* See Treatment Guidelines Based on LDL Cholesterol Level.

of age or sex will similarly decrease the risk of heart disease. Based on these principles, the National Cholesterol Education Program recommends dietary treatment of high blood cholesterol if the LDL cholesterol is greater than 130 in the presence of known heart disease or two of the listed risk factors in the table (Table 3-7). Treatment is also recommended in the absence of any of the known risk factors listed in the table if LDL cholesterol is over 160. Ideally one should attempt to maintain a LDL cholesterol less than 130 mg/dl or maintain a ratio of total cholesterol to HDL cholesterol of less than 4.5. HDL cholesterol levels less than 35 mg/dl represent an increased risk for heart attack.

Although an initial blood cholesterol level can be obtained during any office visit, an elevated value should be confirmed by a repeat analysis performed following an overnight fast. A careful history and physical examination is also needed before considering initiation of diet or drug treatment since certain other medical conditions such as low thyroid function, diabetes mellitus, obstructive liver disease and certain kidney disorders may also produce elevated blood cholesterol levels. Determination of LDL, HDL, and triglyceride levels is also helpful in determining the extent of risk for atherosclerotic vascular disease and helping the physician decide which patients need more aggressive therapy. Specific treatment for high blood triglyceride should be undertaken if this value is above 500 mg/dl since the risk of inflammation of the pancreas (pancreatitis) increases above this level.

The first step in the treatment of persons identified as high or moderate risk is *diet therapy* following the guidelines consistent with those of the American Heart Association. More intensive dietary restrictions may be necessary if the patient fails to respond to initial efforts.

Treatment with cholesterol-lowering drugs should be used only after a careful trial of diet. Cholesterol values change slowly in response to diet, and therefore a three to six month trial of diet modification should be undertaken before considering drug therapy. Some patients are very sensitive to even minor modification in cholesterol and saturated fat intake resulting in prompt decline of blood cholesterol values toward normal. However, because much of body cholesterol is manufactured by the liver and cholesterol levels may be largely genetically determined, diet therapy alone fails in some patients to control hypercholesterolemia.

The importance in reducing cholesterol values has been underscored by the CPPT study which demonstrated that for every 1% reduction in total cholesterol level, a 2% reduction occurred in the rate of heart attack among those men treated with diet and a cholesterol-lowering drug, cholestyramine. As a goal, The National Heart, Lung and Blood Institute Consensus Panel encourages a reduction of blood cholesterol to 180 mg/dl for adults younger

1. **If** your LDL cholesterol level is 130 mg/dl - 159 gm/dl *and* you have either

    A. Known coronary artery disease (previous heart attack, angina pectoris)

    OR

    B. Two of any of the following risk factors:
    - ❏ Male
    - ❏ Parent or sibling with history of coronary heart disease before age 55
    - ❏ Smoke cigarettes
    - ❏ High blood pressure
    - ❏ HDL cholesterol level less than 35 mg/dl
    - ❏ Diabetes
    - ❏ Previous stroke or known hardening of the arteries
    - ❏ Severe obesity (more than 30% overweight)

    then treatment (diet and/or medications) is advised.

2. **If** your LDL cholesterol level is 160 mg/dl or greater, **then** treatment (diet and/or medications) is advised.

than 30 years and to approximately 200 mg/dl for individuals age 30 years or older.

Some physicians feel these target values are unrealistic and that less stringent guidelines should be employed. More importantly, guidelines for blood cholesterol should be individualized for each patient based upon his age and the existence of other active risk factors. For example, patients with established coronary artery disease or those with coronary bypass grafts would require more intensive treatment. In the elderly, since blood cholesterol becomes a less important risk factor, less intense diet or drug therapy would be in order.

Drug treatment for high blood cholesterol.

A variety of medications are available for the treatment of elevated blood cholesterol. It should be stressed, however, that drug therapy should be used only in conjunction with continued efforts at diet modification.

All of the cholesterol-lowering drugs have potential side effects, may have considerable cost, and may have unpleasant side effects. In addition, the long-term safety of these agents over decades of use has not yet been established. Nonetheless, over the shorter term, use of agents such as cholestyramine (Questran®) and gemfibrozil (Lopid®) have been established by the CPPT study and the Helsinki Heart Study as effective means for reducing the risk of heart attack in middle-aged men with elevated blood cholesterol levels. More recently, the introduction of lovastatin (Mevacor®) has been a major addition to the drug treatment armamentarium. This newest cholesterol-lowering drug has proven to be one of the most effective agents presently available. Related drugs are presently under investigation and may be even more potent and possibly safer.

Adverse effects of lovastatin are uncommon but can include rises in blood liver enzymes as well as inflammation of the muscles (myositis). Therefore, patients taking lovastatin should have liver function tests every 4-6 weeks for the first 15 months of treatment and should report any severe muscle aches or pains to their physician. There is also experimental evidence of possible increased risk for development of cataracts, and therefore the manufacturer advises baseline eye examination and yearly examination to monitor for development of cataracts. The actual clinical significance of this risk in humans is as yet unknown.

Blood cholesterol values should be monitored at 4-6 week intervals after instituting drug therapy or after changing treatment dosages.

What role do fish oils play?

Fish oil supplements have gained attention in the popular press as a means for reducing the risk of heart attack. Fish oil supplements contain both cholesterol and saturated fat. As such, they may raise blood LDL and total cholesterol levels. They also contain significant amounts of vitamin A and D which when ingested in large quantities could result in serious toxicity. At this juncture, the data are inconclusive as to whether fish oil supplements provide a protective value against heart attack. Most authorities advise incorporating fish, especially the fatty deep water ocean fish such as salmon, in the diet rather than consuming fish oil capsules. It should also be noted that ingesting large quantities of fish oil may inhibit blood coagulation and thus increase the risk of bleeding in patients taking other anticoagulants (blood thinners).

Elevated blood triglyceride

Elevated blood triglyceride levels have not been associated with cardiovascular risk to the same degree as have elevated blood cholesterol levels. Patients with blood triglyceride levels above 250 mg/dl should be considered for dietary therapy. Triglycerides are increased by excessive calorie intake and especially by increasing calories from carbohydrates such as refined sugars contained in commercial pastry products and candies. Alcohol intake also significantly increases blood triglyceride values. Triglyceride values which remain above 500 mg/dl despite diet warrant drug treatment since these patients are at risk for developing inflammation of the pancreas (pancreatitis).

Nicotinic acid and gemfibrozil are effective and safe triglyceride-lowering drugs. Nicotinic acid may produce flushing and itching initially which can be prevented with a 325 mg. aspirin tablet taken about one hour before the nicotinic acid dose. Nicotinic acid is better tolerated if introduced at low dosage at mealtimes and gradually increased upward in dosage until the desired triglyceride-lowering effect is obtained. Careful monitoring of blood studies for liver inflammation, elevated blood uric acid levels and high blood sugar levels is needed on high dose nicotinic acid therapy.

What is hypertension?

Hypertension is the medical term which describes the presence of high blood pressure. "Hyper" refers to an increase and "tension" refers to force on the artery walls. Therefore hypertension refers to a condition in which the blood pressure force upon the artery walls is increased. Contrary to popular belief, hypertension does not refer to increased excitability or nervousness.

With each heart beat, pressure within the arterial system of the body rises and falls in wave-like fashion. The peak of this wave is termed the systolic pressure, and the bottom of the wave is termed the diastolic pressure. The blood pressure is measured as both systolic and diastolic pressure and expressed as a fraction of systolic pressure over diastolic pressure. Thus, a blood pressure of 120/80 is said aloud as 120 over 80.

Hypertension is a serious risk factor for cardiovascular disease. Patients with uncontrolled hypertension are much more likely to have a heart attack than persons whose blood pressure is normal and most stroke victims have hypertension. However, with control of hypertension, the risk of developing heart attack, stroke, kidney or heart failure is dramatically reduced.

In 95% of patients, no apparent cause can be found for high blood pressure. This form of hypertension, by far the most common, is termed *essential hypertension*. The regulation of blood pressure is a complex interaction of brain and nervous system function, kidney physiology, adrenal gland function, and muscular tone of the venous and arterial circulations. Although the cause of essential hypertension is not known, effective therapy is available.

Occasionally hypertension is the result of a congenital defect such as a constricted aorta (coarctation of the aorta), adrenal gland tumor (pheochromocytoma), an over-active adrenal gland (hyperaldosteronism), underlying kidney disease (nephritis) or narrowed arteries to the kidneys (renovascular hypertension).

How is high blood pressure diagnosed?

Hypertension is diagnosed by a simple blood pressure measurement using an inflatable cuff termed a *sphygmomanometer* (Figure 3-2). Unless the blood pressure reading is very high, a single reading does not constitute the diagnosis of high blood pressure since day-to-day fluctuations may occur. Rather, a finding of increased blood pressure over several measurements is required before the diagnosis of hypertension is established.

Physicians may differ on the precise level at which the diagnosis of hypertension is established, and to some extent, the diagnosis depends upon patient age. Furthermore, the systolic pressure often varies widely throughout the day based upon activity level and other physiologic stresses. The most reliable indicator of high blood pressure is therefore the diastolic pressure. A common classification for diagnosis of high blood pressure is as follows:

1. *Normal blood pressure*: diastolic pressure less than or equal to 90mm. of mercury.
2. *Mild hypertension*: diastolic pressure 90-105 mm. of mercury.
3. *Moderate hypertension*: diastolic pressure 106-115 mm. of mercury.
4. *Severe hypertension*: diastolic pressure greater than 115 mm. of mercury.

Although most patients have mild hypertension, this does not imply that the consequences of untreated hypertension are mild. Over time, even mild hypertension leads to serious consequences. Some people have widely fluctuating blood pressures termed *labile hypertension* which may progress over time to development of sustained hypertension.

Most patients with hypertension do not feel "sick". In fact, they usually feel in good health and the disease is diagnosed only on the basis of a blood pressure measurement. If your physician detects the presence of hypertension, he may well recommend a urinalysis, blood chemistry studies, chest x-ray, electrocardiogram, or echocardiogram (sound wave picture of the heart muscle). This will allow your doctor to determine if injury to certain vital organs has occurred due to high blood pressure and to search for conditions such as kidney or adrenal gland disease, which may be underlying treatable causes of hypertension.

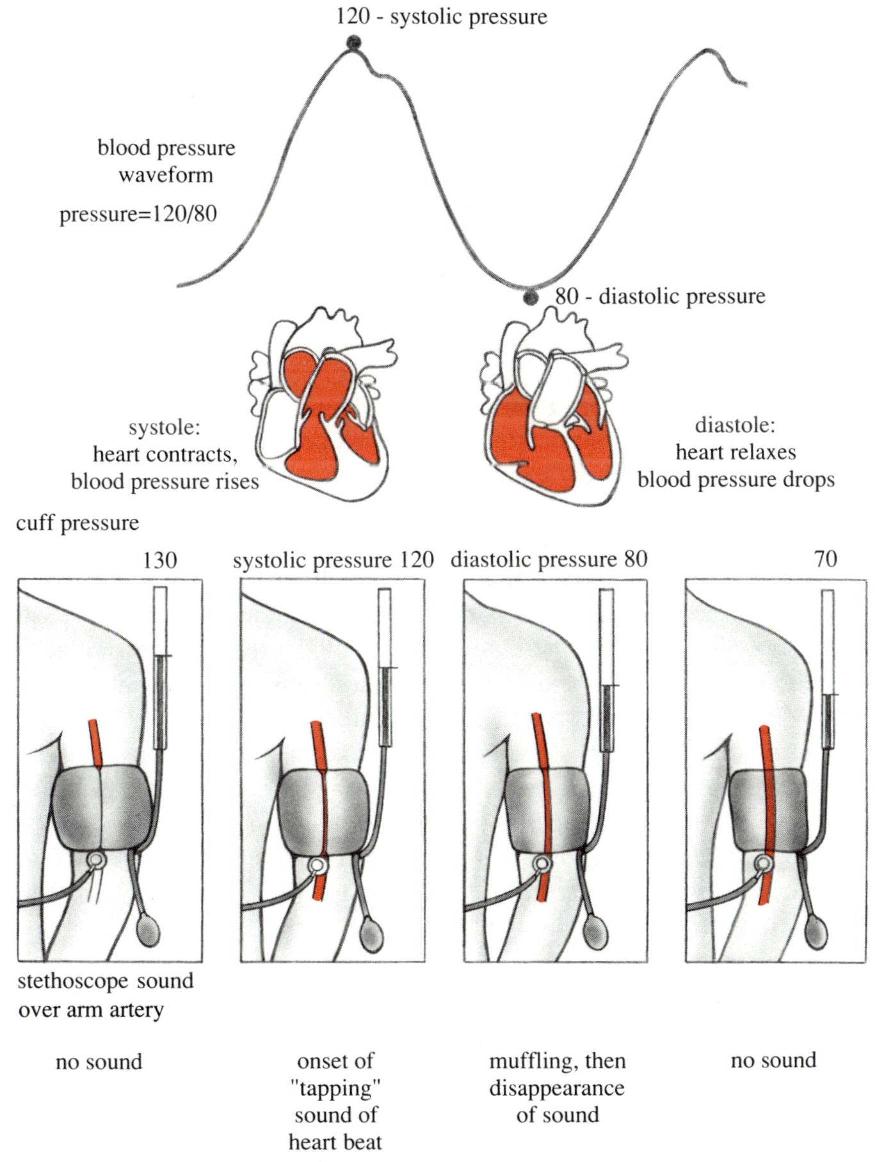

Cardiovascular Disease Risk Factors   63

How is high blood pressure treated?

Treatment of hypertension is one of the most effective means for reducing the risk of heart attack and stroke. Essential hypertension can be effectively treated with diet and medical therapy, but it is important to understand the underlying disorder is not cured. Therefore, therapy and blood pressure monitoring is a life-long process.

Nondrug therapy is often effective for mild forms of hypertension. This includes weight loss, cutting down dietary salt, and regular exercise. In all hypertensive patients, these measures will help reduce the number and dosage of drugs required for treatment of high blood pressure.

Reduction in dietary salt is an important component of nondrug treatment of hypertension. Most Americans consume approximately 10 grams, or 2 teaspoons, of salt (sodium chloride) daily. Present dietary guidelines recommend that we restrict salt consumption to approximately 5 grams, or one teaspoon, daily. Increased amounts of salt in the diet result in an obligatory gain in blood volume which may significantly increase blood pressure in susceptible individuals. There is no present evidence that reduction in salt intake prevents hypertension in persons with normal blood pressure; however, prudent use of salt is a wise measure, especially if a family history of hypertension is present.

One does not need to be a food chemist in order to reduce salt intake to approximately one teaspoon daily. The following guidelines will usually be effective in maintaining salt intake within these ranges: (1) Add little or no salt during food preparation. The use of salt substitutes in sparing quantities may be used if approved by your physician. Salt substitutes are usually potassium chloride preparations which, in the presence of certain medications or kidney disorders, may result in excessive blood potassium levels; (2) Eat fresh meats, vegetables and fruits as much as possible, avoiding canned, processed, or convenience foods; (3) Remove the salt shaker from the table and find alternate spices such as lemon juice or herbs for seasoning; (4) Omit salty foods such as bacon, sausage, potato chips, cottage cheese, pickles and mustard.

Baking soda, monosodium glutamate, luncheon meats and some cereals and puddings are also high sources of salt content. If a diet more stringent in salt restriction is required, consultation with a dietician will be very helpful.

What about exercise and stress relief?

The role of stress in the origin of hypertension and cardiovascular disease is uncertain. Some stress makes life interesting. None of us can avoid stressful situations, and over time it is best to learn when it is important for you to fight back or when it is better to give in. Exercise can also be an excellent form of stress relief and has additional benefits in terms of weight reduction, lowering total and LDL cholesterol levels and increasing HDL cholesterol. Aerobic forms of exercise using rhythmic motions of the arms and legs are best suited to improving cardiovascular conditioning. Isometric exercises that involve straining for prolonged periods of time should generally be avoided. Walking, jogging, bicycling, swimming all provide cardiovascular benefit. Introducing variety into an exercise program and making exercise a family activity increases not only the enjoyment but improves your chances of sticking with a program of regular exercise.

Drug treatment for hypertension.

Fortunately, a wide variety of medications are now available to effectively treat most all cases of hypertension (Table 3-8). However, all medications for hypertension have some side effects, that is, undesirable actions such as dry mouth, fatigability or dizziness. The principal goal of antihypertensive therapy is to find a medication regimen which not only effectively controls blood pressure but also has minimal side effects.

Most high blood pressure medications have some side effects when initially started. It is important not to give up prematurely on these medications since the side effects often disappear with time. However, if the side effects are intolerable, discuss them with your doctor so that an appropriate adjustment in either dosage or use of an alternate medication can be tried. No two people respond to the same medication in the same fashion, and antihypertensive therapy must be highly individualized. Also, different doctors have personal preferences for some antihypertensive medications based upon their previous experiences and their particular approach to the treatment of hypertension. It is important to work closely with your doctor, keep him informed of any side effects, and ask questions as they arise.

In the past, a more standardized format for the treatment of high blood

     MEDICATIONS USED FOR TREATMENT OF HIGH BLOOD PRESSURE

Diuretics

Generic Names	*Common Brand Names*

Thiazide Diuretics

Generic Names	Common Brand Names
chlorothiazide	Diuril®, SK-Chlorothiazide®
chlorthalidone	Hygroton®, Thalitone®
hydrochlorothiazide	Esidrix®, HydroDIURIL®, Oretic®
indapamide	Lozol®
methylclothiazide	Aquatensin®, Enduron®
metolazone	Diulo®, Zaroxolyn®
trichlormethiazide	Metahydrin®, Naqua®

Loop Diuretics

Generic Names	Common Brand Names
bemetanide	Bumex®
ethacrynic acid	Edecrin®
furosemide	Lasix®

Potassium Sparing Diuretics

Generic Names	Common Brand Names
amiloride	Midamor®
spironolactone	Aldactone®
triamterene	Dyrenium®

Sympatholitics

Generic Names	Common Brand Names
clonidine	Catapres®
methyldopa	Aldomet®
guanabenz	Wytensin®

MEDICATIONS USED FOR TREATMENT OF HIGH BLOOD PRESSURE (Cont'd)

Generic Names	*Common Brand Names*
Beta Blockers	
atenolol	Tenormin®
labetalol	Trandate®, Normadyne®
metoprolol	Lopressor®
nadolol	Corgard®
pindolol	Visken®
propanolol	Inderal®, Inderal-LA®
timolol	Blocadren®
Vasodilators	
hydralazine	Apresoline®
minoxidil	Loniten®
prazosin	Minipress®
Angiotensin Converting Inhibitors	
captopril	Capoten®
enalapril	Vasotec®
lisinopril	Zestril®
Combination Agents	
hydrochlorthiazide & spironolactone	Aldactazide®
hydrochlorthiazide & methyldopa	Aldoril®
hydrochlorthiazide & hydralazine	Apresazide®
hydrochlorthiazide & captopril	Capozide®
chlorthalidone & clonidine	Combipres®
bendroflumethazide & nadolal	Corzide®
hydrochlorthiazide & triamterene	Dyazide®
hydrochlorthiazide & propranolol	Inderide®
hydrochlorthiazide & triamterene	Maxzide®
polythiazide & prazosin	Minizide®
chlorthalidone & atenolol	Tenoretic®
hydrochlorthiazide & timolol	Timolide®

pressure was employed termed *step-therapy*. It has generally employed the initial use of a diuretic to which was added, if needed, additional medication such as sympatholytics or vasodilator agents. The treatment of hypertension is once again undergoing significant changes as our understanding of hypertension improves and as new, more effective agents with fewer side effects become available. Step-therapy has now been replaced by a more flexible treatment strategy, designed for the specific needs of each patient.

Diuretics are commonly used in the treatment of hypertension and are commonly referred to as "water pills". They principally act by stimulating an increased excretion of salt and water from the body thereby reducing blood pressure. Some diuretics result in urinary losses of potassium and require the administration of potassium supplements. Thiazide diuretics may increase blood cholesterol levels in some patients to such an extent that a change in antihypertensive therapy is needed. Other diuretics have potassium conserving properties and therefore termed "potassium sparing." Little or no potassium supplementation maybe required with these agents.

Sympatholytics and *beta blockers* comprise a group of drugs which work within the nervous system to reset the body thermostat for high blood pressure, slow heart rate, or reduce the contracting force of the heart muscle.

Vasodilators work by dilating both the artery and venous walls reducing the resistance of blood flow, thus lowering blood pressure.

Angiotensin converting enzyme inhabiters are a new class of agents which inhibit the production of angiotensin, a potent stimulus for high blood pressure. These agents are well tolerated.

Calcium channel blocking agents have also recently been demonstrated effective for the control of hypertension and are now used as initial therapy in some patients with high blood pressure.

What about diabetes?

Although diabetes is not, in the strict sense, a risk factor which can be modified, certainly improved control of diabetes reduces the risk of cardiovascular complications. Reduction of body weight toward ideal, limitation of caloric intake, and regular exercise helps improve the control of diabetes mellitus. Although a cure for diabetes does not exist, close regulation of blood glucose levels can significantly reduce the cardiovascular complications of this illness. Many forms of oral medication termed "oral hypoglycemics" are now available for treatment of diabetes. However, if these agents are poorly tolerated or fail to adequately control blood sugar levels, the use of insulin will be required.

In addition to the dietary guidelines established by the American Heart Association, additional dietary restrictions will likely be required in the presence of diabetes to assist in more effective control. Just as with elevated high blood pressure, high blood sugar levels over time eventually result in progressive atherosclerosis. With good diabetic control, the risk of atherosclerosis can be significantly reduced.

What about smoking?

There is now no question that smoking is one of the most potent risk factors for development of atherosclerosis. When combined with other risk factors such as high blood cholesterol or hypertension, the risks are not merely additive but are multiplied. Therefore if you smoke, you should stop. Your most successful tool in the battle to stop smoking is a sincere desire to quit. The use of a nicotine resin gum (Nicorette®) can significantly increase your chances of breaking the habituation link in the smoking habit. But just as with weight loss, the key to smoking cessation is to stay off cigarettes. Your desire and commitment to smoking cessation is vital.

Summary

Understanding cardiovascular risk factors is an essential step in the treatment and prevention of cardiovascular disease. Many of these risk factors are modifiable, that is, can be treated with diet, medication or lifestyle changes. The resulting decrease in risk for heart attack, stroke or other ravages of cardiovascular disease can be dramatic and rewarding since the presence of multiple risk factors is not like adding them together but more like multiplying them together. With few exceptions, these risk factors can now be effectively modified, but the most important factor in this success equation is *you.*

Chapter Four

Congestive Heart Failure, Heart Rhythm Disturbances, and Valvular Heart Disease

CONGESTIVE HEART FAILURE

What is congestive heart failure?

The term "heart failure" is a frightening term when heard for the first time but actually describes a rather common cardiac condition. Congestive heart failure (CHF) refers to a condition in which the heart muscle is in a weakened state. As the heart weakens, the cardiac chambers gradually dilate. In the early stages of this disorder, the progressive dilation actually helps improve contracting strength of the heart muscle. However, as the muscle weakens further, the dilation then serves to hinder heart muscle contraction resulting in a progressive rise of blood pressure within the cardiac chambers.

These rising cardiac pressures produce increased blood pressure within the draining veins of the lung. High venous lung pressures cause seepage of fluid from the lung capillaries into the tissue spaces of the lung itself producing symptoms of shortness of breath and fatigue. Generalized fluid retention commonly occurs and may be noticeable as ankle swelling.

What causes congestive heart failure?

Congestive heart failure is the end result of any disease process which either overburdens the heart muscle or actually damages heart muscle tissue (Figure 4-1). Therefore, congestive heart failure may be the consequence of previous heart attack, overwork of the heart from high blood pressure or valvular heart disease, or direct heart muscle injury due to alcohol abuse. Rarely, congestive heart failure results from infection of the heart with a virus or as an inherited disorder.

How is congestive heart failure diagnosed?

Symptoms of congestive heart failure such as fatigue and shortness of breath are often important clues to the initial diagnosis. Physical examination may reveal evidence of fluid within lung tissues (rales) or an abnormal gallop rhythm of the heart.

More commonly, however, additional studies are required to confirm the diagnosis of congestive heart failure. The chest x- ray is often very helpful in initial diagnostic evaluation. Because congestive heart failure results in weakening of the heart muscle and progressive cardiac chamber dilation, evidence of cardiac enlargement on chest x-ray is an important clue to the diagnosis of congestive heart failure. Elevated blood pressures within the cardiac chambers are often reflected as engorgement of the draining pulmonary veins, another finding which can be detected by chest x-ray examination.

More precise information as to heart muscle chamber size and contracting function can be obtained by either echocardiography or nuclear cardiac testing. Echocardiography employs high frequency sound waves which are reflected from the interior of the heart chambers resulting in a cross-sectional image of the moving heart muscle (Figure 4-2). The reflected sound waves can also be further analyzed to gain information regarding blood flow velocity in a technique called Doppler echocardiography. Echocardiography has the distinct advantage of being entirely noninvasive and using no radiation to obtain an image. It may be repeated several times over the course of therapy in order to determine if improvements in cardiac chamber size and contracting function have occurred. This gives your doctor important insights into the response of your heart to treatment.

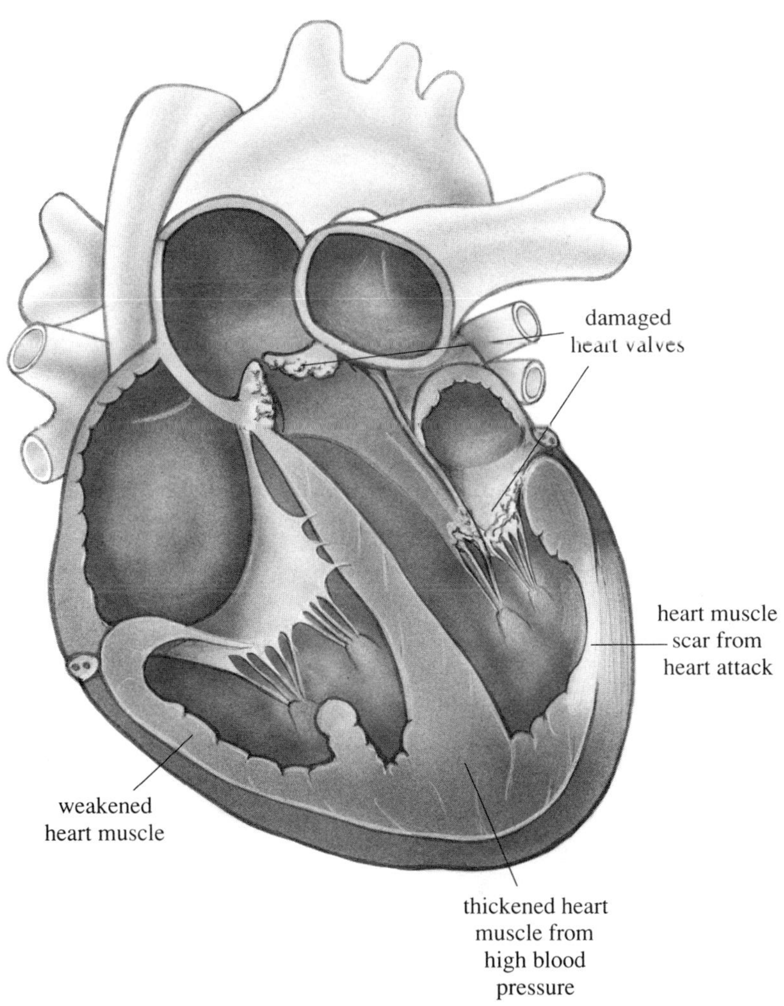
damaged
heart valves
heart muscle
scar from
heart attack
weakened
heart muscle
thickened heart
muscle from
high blood
pressure

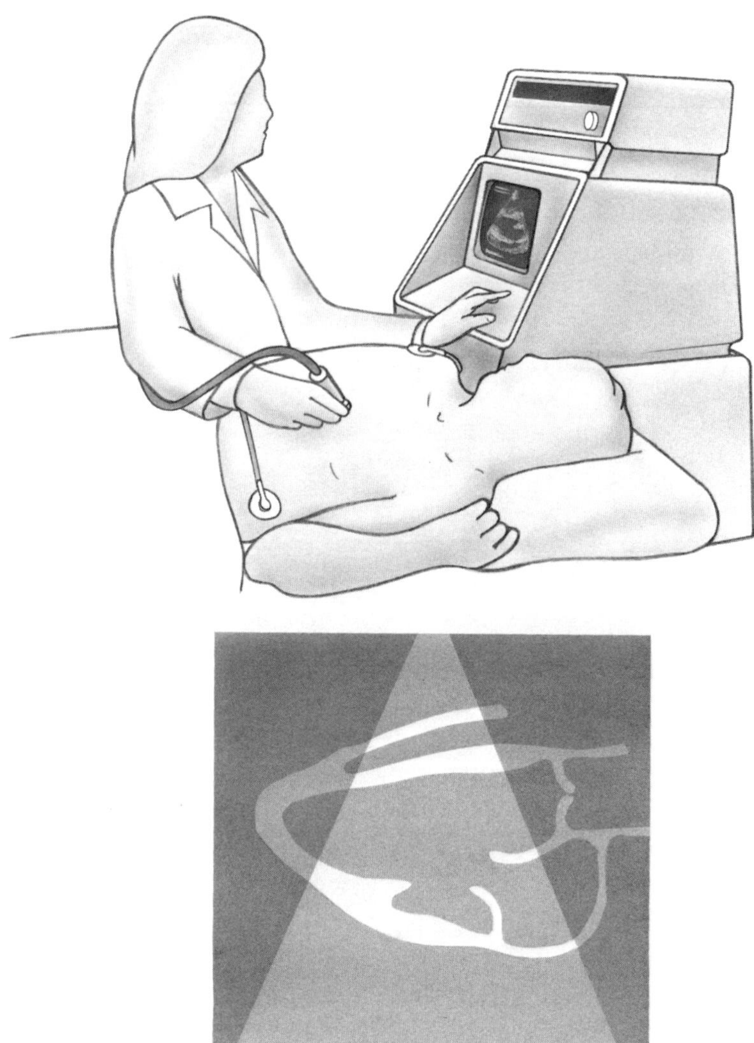

cross-sectional image
of the left ventricle
and mitral valve

Another technique to measure heart muscle contracting function is the nuclear gated blood pool scan, also called a MUGA Scan. In this noninvasive technique, a small injection of a radioisotope is given in an arm vein. The pumping action of the heart muscle can then be evaluated with a nuclear camera and a picture of the pumping chamber obtained. Precise calculation of the blood volume ejected with each beat (ejection fraction) can be determined by this technique.

Finally, heart catheterization gives additional insights into the extent of heart muscle abnormality and allows direct measurement of pressures within the heart chambers.

How is congestive heart failure treated?

Treatment of congestive heart failure largely depends upon the precise cause of the disorder in a given patient. For example, if high blood pressure is producing an increased work load on the heart muscle, then treatment directed toward lowering blood pressure to normal values is very useful in alleviating congestive heart failure. Other times, the precise cause for congestive heart failure cannot be easily remedied, such as heart muscle damage due to previous heart attack or muscle damage from long-standing hypertension. In these circumstances, medications are very useful in improving heart muscle contraction and in reducing heart chamber pressures toward normal values, thereby reducing the work burden on the weakened heart.

Digitalis derivatives such as digoxin (Lanoxin®) help improve heart muscle contracting strength. Diuretics such as furosemide (Lasix®) help the kidneys excrete excessive fluid from the lungs and circulatory system, reducing heart pressures toward normal values. Recent scientific studies have demonstrated that use of angiotensin converting enzyme inhibitors (ACE inhibitors) such as captopril (Capoten®) and enalopril (Vasotec®) are effective in reducing the resistance to blood outflow from the cardiac chambers thus improving not only the ability of the heart to pump blood forward , but may give some patients with congestive heart failure improved survival. ACE inhibitors may also significantly improve the work and exercise capacity of patients with congestive heart failure. Thus, in some circumstances both longevity and quality of life can be enhanced. Like all potent circulatory medications, angiotensin converting enzyme inhibitors have possible side effects and are not indicated in the treatment of all patients with congestive heart failure.

Another important advancement in the treatment of patients with severe congestive heart failure is amrinone (Inocor®). This agent is usually reserved for patients unresponsive to other measures and is given as an intravenous infusion over a period of several days. Amrinone acts to increase the strength of heart muscle contraction thus giving the heart and circulatory system a temporary boost. This boost, however, can reestablish the delicate equilibrium of the circulatory system and may provide the patient with several months of improved exercise capacity and reduced symptoms.

In advanced congestive heart failure, heart transplantation is now an accepted and effective means of treatment for certain patients. Although initial transplant survival rates were low, these statistics have been dramatically improved with the advent of cyclosporin A. This medication helps reduce the risk of heart transplant rejection and has greatly improved the long-term survival of heart transplant patients. Unfortunately, one of the greatest limitations to heart transplant at this time remains the relative lack of suitable donors.

What dietary restrictions are needed for treatment of congestive heart failure?

One of the most important dietary restrictions required in the treatment of congestive heart failure is that of sodium restriction. Sodium, as contained in ordinary table salt, is a basic constituent of all body fluids. As such, it must be dissolved within the body by a required amount of body fluid. Excessive intake of salt therefore results in a mandatory gain in body content. Because congestive heart failure is worsened by excessive blood and tissue fluid retention, reduction of dietary salt intake is essential in treatment (Table 4-1).

ABNORMALITIES OF HEART RHYTHM

What is normal heart rhythm?

Normal heart rhythm is under the control of a series of delicately timed electrical clocks within the heart muscle. Special electrical heart nerve fibers send the electric signals from these clocks to all areas of heart muscle to initiate contraction. In a normally beating heart, a small electric clock at the top of the right atrium, termed the sinoatrial node, spontaneously discharges electrical pulses approximately every 8/10 of a second during normal resting heart action. This electrical activity initially spreads through the upper heart chambers or atria, causing them to contract and empty blood into the lower receiving pumping chambers, the ventricles. The orderly sequential contraction of the atria and ventricles is termed normal sinus rhythm.

Table 4-1 **TIPS ON CUTTING SALT (SODIUM) INTAKE**

❑ Don't add salt at the table. Use an herb shaker for seasoning.

❑ Avoid high sodium seasonings: soy sauce, MSG (monosodium glutamate), steak sauce.

❑ Don't use packaged foods if the words salt or sodium are listed near the start of the ingredient list.

❑ Avoid salty foods such as salted snack foods, pickles, canned soups, cured meats.

❑ Eat fresh meats, vegetables and fruits as much as possible.

❑ Salt substitutes may be used in sparring quantities if approved by your physician. Salt substitutes are usually potassium-rich, which in the presence of certain medications or kidney disorders, may result in excessive blood potassium levels.

What are the symptoms of abnormal heart rhythm?

Abnormal heart rhythm may be entirely without symptoms. However often certain sensations or experiences occur as a result of an altered heart rhythm, or arrhythmia.

The most common of these is the sense of palpitation. Palpitation refers to the subjective sense of abnormality of heart beat. This may be perceived as a sense of rapid heart action, a sense of excessively slow heart action, a sense of extra or skipped heart beats, or a sense of "fluttering" in the chest. Bradycardia is the medical term used to describe a slow heart beat and derives its meaning from brady, meaning slow, and cardia, pertaining to the heart. Similarly, tachycardia, means fast heart beat.

More serious disturbances of heart rhythm may actually impair blood flow to the brain causing a momentary loss of consciousness or in medical terms, syncope. Syncope may be one of the initial manifestations of an underlying disorder of heart rhythm.

Premature ventricular contractions, or PVC for short, are one of the most common heart rhythm disturbances. Premature ventricular contractions occur when an area in the ventricle spontaneously discharges its electrical activity prematurely, out of sequence from normal sinus rhythm. This results in a weak and forceless heart beat which is followed thereafter by a brief pause. The next beat following the pause is more forceful than a normal cardiac beat producing a sense of sudden thrusting or pounding within the chest. PVC's may cause a sense of heart "hesitation" or a sense of "skipped heart beat". In actuality, this is a premature beat followed by a more forceful beat.

Premature ventricular contractions are extremely common occurrences and occur daily in entirely normal hearts. However, in a small select group of patients, PVC's pose a risk for more serious or life-threatening irregularities of cardiac rhythm. Some patients who fall into this high risk category are those with severe congestive heart failure or those with advanced coronary artery disease. More severe electrical instability will produce repetitive runs of premature ventricular contractions termed ventricular tachycardia.

Palpitations may also be the result of abnormally rapid rhythm from the atrial chambers. These episodes typically occur and disappear with abrupt onset and other than for an unpleasant sense of rapid heart beat generally do not produce dangerous symptoms. This rhythm disorder, because of its abrupt on and off character, is termed paroxysmal atrial tachycardia.

Bradycardia describes an abnormally slow heart rate. If severe slowing in heart rhythm is present, insertion of a permanent pacemaker will be required. Pacemaker insertion is accomplished by placing a small electrical pulse generator beneath the skin of the left shoulder region. A small plastic-coated electrode is then introduced into the subclavian vein beneath the collar bone and advanced under x-ray guidance to the tip of the right ventricle. The pacing electrode is then connected to the pacemaker pulse generator. Sometimes a second electrode lead is also placed in the right atrium. The pacemaker generator continuously and automatically monitors cardiac rhythm and in the event of a pause or slowing of heart rhythm below a predetermined rate, the pacemaker will then discharge a small and imperceptible electrical impulse into the pacing electrode stimulating the heart to contract.

How are arrhythmias treated?

Some forms of heart rhythm disturbance can be readily corrected by avoiding or treating aggravating factors such as excessive coffee intake, emotional or physical stress, overactive thyroid gland function, or abnormalities in blood potassium level.

Other times, specific medications called antiarrhythmic agents are required. The specific medication used is a highly individualized decision for each patient. Generally medications such as digoxin, verapamil or beta blockers are employed for treatment of paroxysmal atrial tachycardia whereas other agents such as quinidine, procainamide, or flecainide are used for treatment of ventricular arrhythmias. The choice of a specific agent depends upon the type and severity of the patient's rhythm disorder as well as any associated cardiac conditions such as congestive heart failure which might be worsened by some antiarrhythmic medication. Most importantly, all antiarrhythmic agents have some undesirable side effects. These side effects may be rather mild such as nausea and tremors or more serious side effects such as an aggravation of the underlying rhythm disturbance (proarrhythmic effect). Therefore, a very careful analysis of the risk versus benefit of antiarrhythmic therapy is needed before embarking upon any course of antiarrhythmic treatment.

Many antiarrhythmic drugs require periodic monitoring of blood levels or EKG's to make certain the medication is within safe and therapeutic ranges.

How are heart rhythm abnormalities diagnosed?

Since the electrocardiogram is an electrical measure of the heart rhythm system, it is of fundamental importance in diagnosis of cardiac arrhythmias.

Unfortunately, many disorders of heart rhythm are episodic in nature, and therefore, a single EKG may miss the precise moment a rhythm disturbance occurs. A 24-hour continuous electrocardiogram recording called a Holter monitor test may well be required to determine the type and severity of rhythm disturbances present (Figure 4-3). This small portable electrocardiogram machine is worn from a belt suspended around the shoulder or waist and is connected to skin electrodes on the chest and trunk. The heart rhythm is continuously recorded on electromagnetic cassette tapes which can then be played back at a later time, reproducing the entire 24-hour record of heart rhythm. The patient is usually asked to record symptoms and activities in a diary booklet provided at the time the Holter is applied. This allows correlation between the EKG Holter tracings and any significant symptoms. Holter monitoring may clarify the arrhythmia diagnosis and is also a useful means by which the response to antiarrhythmic therapy can be measured. Holter monitor data may indicate adequate control of the heart rhythm disturbance or may point to a need to change drug type or dosage.

VALVULAR HEART DISEASE

What is valvular heart disease?

Valvular heart disease occurs when a heart valve fails to operate in proper fashion (Figure 4-4). Typically this occurs when the valve either fails to open fully, a condition termed valvular stenosis, or when the valve fails to close properly resulting in back leakage or regurgitation of blood through the valve leaflets. Normal heart valve leaflets are thin, pliable structures which open fully and allow unimpeded passage of blood then promptly close and seal tightly, preventing the regurgitation of blood. Rheumatic fever or valve infection may result in scarring or degeneration of the valve tissue leading to valvular stenosis or regurgitation. Other times valve tissue may degenerate, thicken, and deposit calcium as a result of the aging process.

Another common disorder of heart valve function is that of mitral valve

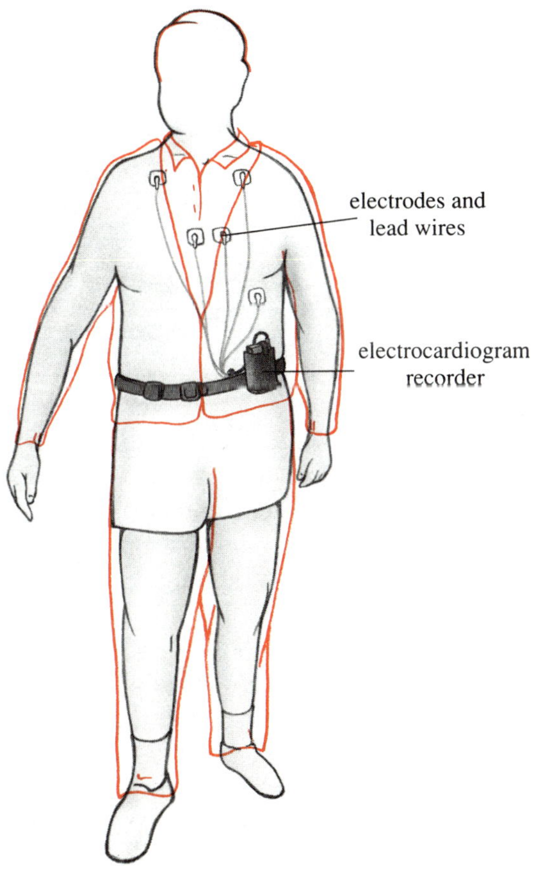
electrodes and
lead wires
electrocardiogram
recorder

prolapse. Normally, the mitral valve closes in a tight "V" configuration. In mitral valve prolapse the leaflets bulge or prolapse backward toward the left atrium as the valve attempts to close. This may result in back leakage of blood from the left ventricle into the left atrium. However, many times no mitral valve regurgitation occurs and only a clicking noise is evident during examination as the valve leaflets prolapse into a closed configuration.

Mitral valve prolapse is best thought of as a slight variation in an otherwise normal heart. Although mitral valve prolapse may produce fleeting episodes of chest discomfort or may produce arrhythmias, such as PVC's, rarely is it a serious threat to health. Probably the most serious problem related to mitral valve prolapse is that of progressive and severe mitral regurgitation which fortunately occurs in only a small percentage of patients with this disorder.

How is valvular heart disease diagnosed?

As with all cardiac disorders, history and physical examination provide important clues to the diagnosis of valvular heart disease. One of the most common findings on examination is that of a murmur. A murmur simply describes an abnormal squirting sound within the heart chambers.

Typically, when blood flows through a cardiac valve, no sound is made other than the soft closing sound of the valve leaflets. This results in the typical "lub-dub" sound of the heart beat. However, if a valve fails to open fully or if a valve allows regurgitation of blood, a squirting noise or murmur is produced. This is much like putting one's finger over the tip of a garden hose causing the water to squirt through the small opening.

Not all heart murmurs, however, are a reflection of valvular heart disease. Occasionally an abnormal communication between heart chambers such as an atrial or ventricular septal defect will cause a murmur. Other times a heart murmur may occur in an entirely normal heart simply due to increased blood flow or due to a thin chest wall which allows enhanced detection of normal blood flow sounds. This is analogous to the gurgling noise a rain-swollen stream might make due to increased water flow. These so-called "innocent murmurs" are common in young children because of a child's relatively high cardiac output and thin chest wall.

Beyond physical examination, echocardiography with Doppler study is an indispensable part of the evaluation of valvular heart disease. Because

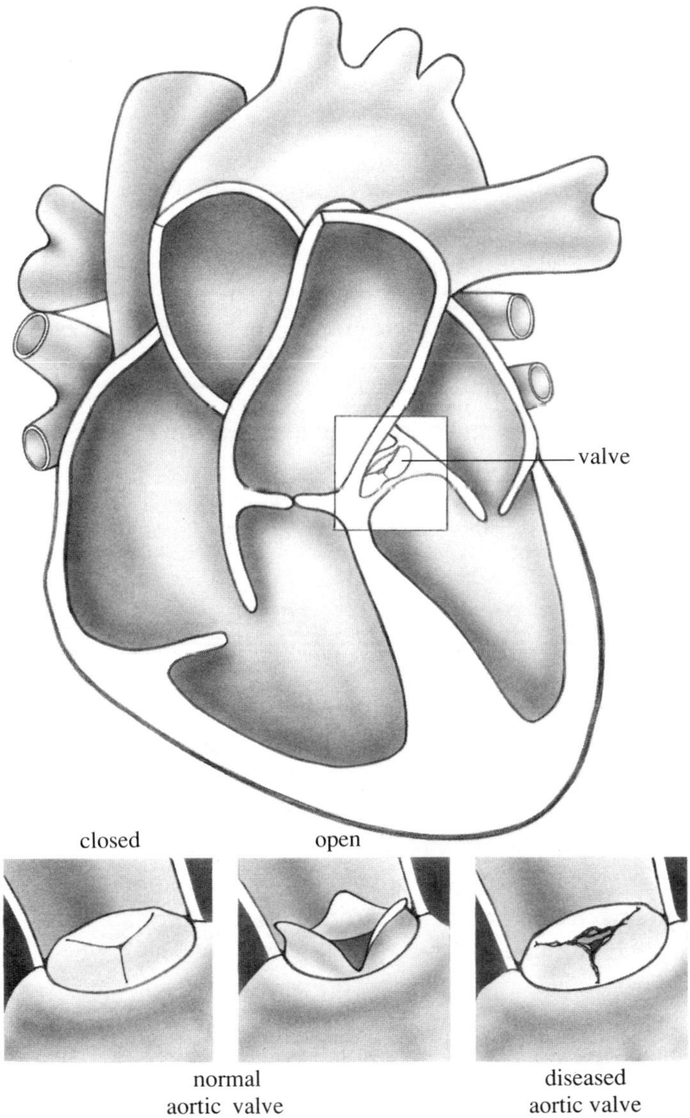

Valvular Heart Disease: Deformity or scarring of a heart valve may prevent normal opening and closure leading to valvular obstruction (stenosis) or leakage (regurgitation).

echocardiography allows the physician to see a cross-sectional image of the heart valves, disturbances in valve architecture, mobility and closure can be detected. In addition, blood flow velocity patterns can be carefully analyzed through the use of Doppler echocardiography. The Doppler technique reflects high frequency sound waves from the blood flowing through a valve orifice allowing measurement of blood flow velocity. A great deal of information can be obtained from this Doppler data including information regarding valve opening size,pressure difference across the valve orifice, and the extent to which valve leakage is present.

In addition to analysis of valve function itself, echocardiography allows the cardiologist to accurately measure heart chamber size and function, thus giving important clues as to the overall effects of valve leakage or stenosis on heart muscle action. This information, in conjunction with other data such as symptoms, is often crucial in determining whether heart valve replacement is needed.

Heart catheterization also provides detailed and precise information regarding valve function and also allows examination of the coronary arteries to detect any associated coronary blockage.

How is valvular heart disease treated?

The heart itself has an amazing ability to adapt to abnormalities in valve function. In mild and moderate cases of valvular regurgitation or stenosis, activity restrictions and medication often suffice for treatment. Medications such as those used for treatment of congestive heart failure are often used. In addition, restriction in activity is important for certain valvular abnormalities.

Aortic valve narrowing, aortic stenosis, when present in moderate or severe degree requires restriction from vigorous physical activity. This is important since exercise greatly increases the pumping demand on the main left ventricular chamber. Because aortic stenosis prevents the rapid emptying of the main left ventricular pumping chamber, overexertion can lead to serious consequence and even complete circulatory collapse. Similarly, avoidance of heavy physical exertion is advised in cases of significant valvular regurgitation or mitral valve stenosis.

Mitral valve prolapse is a common disorder and may occur in approximately 10-15% of all females. However, except in the most severe instances of prolapse, this disorder is best thought of as a slight variation in an

      **A MECHANICAL AORTIC VALVE IMPLANT:
THE ST. JUDE VALVE**

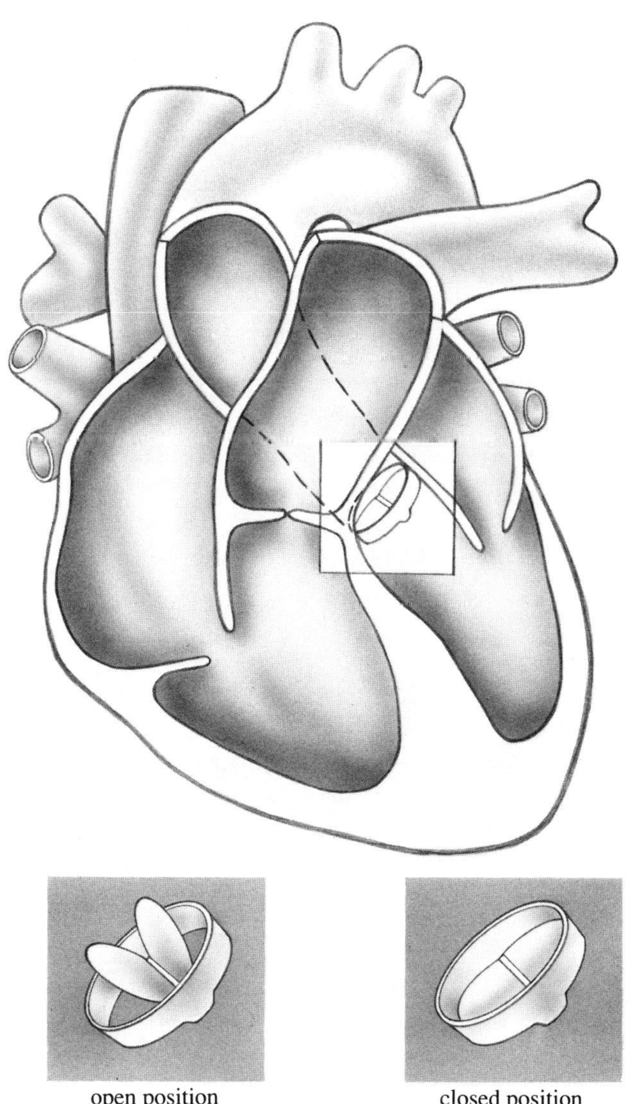

otherwise normal heart. Occasionally mitral valve prolapse can produce fleeting episodes of chest discomfort or palpitations which may require specific medication for symptom relief. Beta blockers are commonly employed in this regard.

All abnormal valve structures are at risk for infection if bacteria enter the bloodstream. Bacteria tend to deposit in areas of abnormal blood flow within the circulation. Thus, the altered blood flow through an abnormal heart valve poses an on-going risk to infection, termed endocarditis, during dental work or surgical procedures. Antibiotics given before and after these procedures in accordance with the recommendations of The American Heart Association greatly reduce the risk of valve infection.

If valve function is severely abnormal, surgical replacement of the valve will often be necessary. This is accomplished by surgical removal of the diseased valve tissue and implantation of either a mechanical or tissue valve (Figure 4-5). Valves of mechanical design employ either a moving disc occluder or a ball-in-cage mechanism. They offer the specific advantage of substantially improved durability as compared with tissue valves. However, as a drawback, lifelong anticoagulation therapy is necessary and this may not be suitable for certain patients. An alternate form of artificial heart valve is the tissue valve. Tissue valves are constructed either from a pig aortic valve or from the membrane pericardial sac of a calf heart. The tissue is then specially treated with gluteraldehyde which acts like a tanning agent to turn the leaflets into a soft pliable leather-like material. The treated valve tissue is then sewn by the manufacturer onto a strut and ring apparatus. The completed valve is then ready for implantation.

Tissue valves have the advantage of, in some circumstances, avoiding the need for long-term anticoagulant therapy. However, over time tissue valves tend to degenerate forming calcium deposits and small leaflet tears such that 10 to 15 years post implantation many tissue valves demonstrate significant degeneration.

Living heart valves have also been implanted as substitutes for diseased valves. This technique, termed homograft valve transplantation, has not gained widespread use or acceptance to date in the United States. The logistic difficulties in obtaining fresh valve tissue from cadaver donors and preserving this valve tissue for subsequent implantation has proven difficult. Therefore, in the United States, surgical replacement with a prosthetic valve or repair of the defective heart valve is employed much more commonly than is homograft valve implantation.

Recently, increasing interest has been given to surgical techniques designed to repair the defective heart valve. Open surgical ultrasound debridement of the aortic valve has been recently reported. This technique involves the use of a small probe emitting high frequency ultrasound waves. The ultrasound probe is used to dislodge calcified nodules from the aortic valve rendering the valve leaflets more pliable. Another open surgical technique is that of mitral commissurotomy in which the narrowed opening of a mitral valve scarred by rheumatic fever is opened by surgical incision along the closure lines or commissures of the valve. Yet another important surgical technique of valve repair is that of mitral valvuloplasty which is employed in the treatment of severe mitral regurgitation due to mitral valve prolapse. In this technique, the redundant floppy mitral valve tissue is "gathered up" in an attempt to reshape the mitral valve and prevent valvular regurgitation. Sometimes this may not produce an adequate repair and necessitate proceeding onward to complete valve replacement during the same surgical procedure.

The most recent development in treatment of valvular stenosis is that of balloon valvuloplasty. This technique involves advancement of a balloon catheter across a narrowed valve followed by a period of brief balloon inflation. The balloon catheter is advanced into the heart usually from the femoral artery of the groin in a fashion analogous to that employed for routine cardiac catheterization. It remains yet to be determined how useful this treatment will be in the overall management of patients with valvular stenosis. At this time, most practitioners of balloon valvuloplasty reserve the method for patients who are otherwise poor surgical candidates due to advanced age, poor overall heart function, or because of associated illness known to increase surgical risk of valve replacement or repair.

All artificial heart valves, diseased heart valves, or valves that have undergone repair techniques require protection with antibiotics before and after dental work. Artificial (prosthetic) heart valves are at especially high risk for infection, and therefore, more vigorous antibiotic prophylaxis protocols have been recommended for protection of prosthetic heart valves during surgery or dental procedures. It is advisable for all patients with prosthetic valves to wear an identification bracelet describing the name of the valve replaced and the type of prosthetic valve implanted. Similarly, for those patients with prosthetic valves requiring anticoagulation, this should be also clearly marked on their identification bracelet. Generally, a wallet I.D. card is given to the patient with a prosthetic heart valve following surgery and contains complete information regarding the valve type, valve serial number and other important identifying data.

Chapter Five

Preparing For Recovery And Hospital Discharge

Coping with heart disease.

The diagnosis of heart disease often leaves you with a variety of emotions including that of fear, resentment and anxiety. These are common feelings and are experienced to some degree by all heart patients. You may feel angry and frustrated or as if you are living on borrowed time. You become increasingly aware of all discomforts within your chest such that the tiniest discomfort brings back concerns of impending heart attack or catastrophe.

You may have spells of feeling "blue" or "crippled" and on days there may seem to be no hope ahead. You may find yourself short-tempered and irritable at the slightest provocation. These feelings and changes in moods are a normal part of adaption following the diagnosis of heart disease. Sharing these with your family, friends and doctor helps lessen the stress provoked by these emotions. With the passage of time these feelings do disappear, but they can often be uncomfortable and worrisome in the meantime.

Heart disease also affects the family of each patient. Children or teenagers may find themselves feeling guilty as if they were responsible for your health problems. If you were hospitalized in the Coronary Care Unit or have undergone coronary bypass graft surgery or coronary angioplasty, your family, even though they may have not shown it, was clearly worried and frightened by the experience. It is best to talk about these feelings with your family and bring them out into the open.

You may also be concerned about your ability to return to a normal life and to engage in normal sexual and recreational activities. If you are employed, you may have legitimate concerns about your ability to return to work and the economic impact of these changes on your family budget.

The good news is that most patients can return to many of their previous activities and return to work. Each case is clearly individualized, though, and depends upon the degree to which the heart circulation is impaired, or in the case of heart attack, the extent to which heart muscle damage has occurred. A program of rehabilitation, whether carried out at home or in a program of supervised cardiac rehabilitation, is a positive step toward return to an active and fulfilling life.

What precautions are necessary?

If you've undergone cardiac catheterization, coronary angioplasty, coronary bypass graft surgery or if you sustained a heart attack, certain general precautions are necessary in the initial days following hospital discharge.

Following cardiac catheterization or coronary angioplasty, the arterial puncture site in the groin should be protected from vigorous exertion, prolonged walking, or straining maneuvers which might provoke bleeding. The site should be kept clean and dry and covered with a band-aid during this period of time. Bruising is not uncommon and is caused by several tablespoons of blood that seep out around the catheters when they are in the artery of the groin. Bruising may spread over the surface of the thigh and even up onto the front of the stomach area. This should not cause alarm and gradually will be reabsorbed over the next 2-3 weeks during which time the blood by-products will be remanufactured into new blood cells. However, if progressive pain or swelling in the groin occurs, this may be a sign of infection or of a blood pocket overlying the puncture site called a *hematoma* or *pseudoaneurysm*. Should you notice these complaints, be certain and report immediately to your doctor for re-examination. Similarly, any signs of redness, fever, wound drainage or red streaking of the skin at the catheterization or angioplasty site should be reported immediately.

As a part of the natural healing process following coronary angioplasty, scar tissue develops on the interior of the vessel and may result in progressive renarrowing of the coronary artery. This process, termed restenosis, may cause a return in anginal symptoms. The scar formation occurs within the first six months following coronary angioplasty and is rare thereafter. If you notice a recurrence of your angina pain following coronary angioplasty, be certain to report again to your cardiologist or family physician in order that he can re-evaluate your status and determine whether renarrowing of the dilation site is a possible cause for these symptoms.

Following hospital discharge for heart attack or coronary bypass graft surgery, you will find that usual physical activities may leave you feeling drained and exhausted. This is a natural response since the period of bed rest during hospitalization results in significant physical deconditioning. It is important to continue your home activities in the same pace as those at time of hospital discharge and to gradually, and with realistic expectations, progressively increase your activity thereafter.

The heart is surrounded and supported by a thin membrane sac called the pericardium. The pericardium is richly supplied by nerves and becomes inflamed to some degree in all patients who have had coronary bypass graft surgery or sustained a heart attack. If this inflammation becomes severe, it may result in sharp, stabbing pains in the chest which are increased during deep breathing, while coughing or when lying down. This problem, called *Dressler's syndrome* or *pericarditis*, is a natural response of the membrane sac to coronary bypass graft surgery or heart attack. Medications to reduce inflammation can be prescribed by your doctor and then gradually discontinued as the inflammation subsides.

Following coronary bypass graft surgery your chest incision and leg wounds should be carefully inspected for any signs of infection such as redness, swelling or drainage. Any signs of infection or any fever should be reported promptly to your doctor. When the wound margins have sealed together, your doctor will allow you to begin tub baths or showers. It is important to move carefully in and out of the tub or shower since you might find yourself weak or sore during these maneuvers. Use warm water and wash gently. Be certain to avoid hot water which might make you feel faint or dizzy.

Elastic or support stockings supplied for the patient following coronary bypass graft surgery should be worn for the first several weeks while at home. This helps reduce leg swelling which usually occurs to some degree following removal of the saphenous vein for bypass grafting. Excessive swelling may interfere with wound healing and increase the risk of infection. When possible during rest periods, sit with your leg elevated to help further reduce tissue swelling. Initially you will find it necessary to ask your family to assist in putting on and removing your stockings.

Your breastbone takes approximately 4-6 weeks to heal following coronary bypass graft surgery. During this period of time, you may notice occasional "clicking" since the breastbone, like any healing bone, is somewhat unstable during this period of time. During the first 4-6 weeks, avoid driving yourself in an automobile and limit trips to necessary travel since any accident or sudden stop might bump your chest and reinjure the sternum.

Be certain and take adequate time for rest following heart attack or coronary bypass graft surgery. A rest period for 20-30 minutes in the mid morning and late afternoon is very helpful. Visitation should be kept to those of immediate family and close friends since keeping up a conversation and relating the events of your illness and hospitalization is an exhausting experience for all patients.

After a heart attack or coronary bypass graft surgery, it is a good idea to keep a log of your daily weights for the first 4-6 weeks since any gain of 2-3 pounds over several days indicates excessive retention of body fluids. This should be reported to your doctor so that changes in your diet or medication can be undertaken.

If an occasional drink has been your custom prior to heart attack or surgery, you can continue this in moderation during the recovery period. However, you should limit the amount of alcohol to no greater than 2 ounces per day which would be the amount of alcohol in two 12 ounce beers, 6 ounces of wine or 2 ounces of whiskey. Alcohol should not be combined with pain medication, tranquilizers or sleeping pills.

What about exercise?

A program of progressive physical activity is a cornerstone in the rehabilitation of each cardiac patient. Exercise helps the cardiac patient in a variety of ways. First, bed rest and immobilization during hospitalization results in a loss of 15-20% of normal muscular strength. Initially you will find that activities of daily life such as brushing your teeth, combing your hair and dressing may produce a sense of fatigue and shortness of breath.

Second, exercise is an important step in reducing risk factors for future heart disease. A program of regular exercise reduces body weight toward ideal and has a favorable effect in lowering blood cholesterol and triglyceride levels.

Additionally, exercise aids in the control of other cardiac risk factors such as hypertension, diabetes, and can significantly help in a program of smoking cessation.

Third, regular physical activity helps the arms, legs and lungs work as more efficient partners with the heart. This results in more efficient use of oxygen and reduces the overall work load on the heart. The net result is the ability to perform greater levels of exercise at lower levels of cardiac work load.

An exercise program for the cardiac patient should be individually prescribed. Exercise should be limited to those levels of heart rate and blood pressure which do not provoke excessive fatigue, chest discomfort, heart rhythm disturbances or abnormalities in blood pressure. Oftentimes it is necessary to perform an exercise treadmill test in order that an "exercise prescription" can be formulated outlining the type and intensity of exercise best suited for each individual.

Some general guidelines, however, apply to most all patients (Table 5-1). First, any program of physical activity should be started gradually. Following hospital discharge, it is best to maintain activity levels similar to those in the hospital. Most household activities are permitted including self-care and light household activities. However, you should avoid making beds, washing and hanging out clothes, or floor scrubbing since these activities often involve significant physical exertion.

A program of walking is often best suited to the cardiac patient. This form of exercise, called "aerobic exercise", involves the repetitive to and fro motion of large groups of muscles. Aerobic exercise is an excellent way to condition the cardiovascular system. A program of walking 20-30 minutes every other day will result in a significant conditioning effect over a period of 4-6 weeks (Table 5-2). You should first start at a slow pace, taking specific care not to exceed the target heart rate set by your doctor. This target heart rate has been determined for your individual circumstance in order to produce benefit from exercise yet reduce the risk of over-exertion. Your target heart rate can be monitored by counting your pulse (Figure 5-1). It is usually easiest to obtain an accurate pulse rate from one of the large arteries in the neck called the carotid artery. Rest your thumb on the chin and with your fingers you can feel the pulse rate along the side of the neck. Your pulse can also be counted at the wrist or elbow or by placing your hand over the apex of the heart beat.

Stop periodically during your walking program to count your pulse rate. Count for only ten seconds and multiply the result by six to obtain the pulse rate per minute. Since the heart rate decelerates rapidly after stopping exercise, counting for longer than ten seconds results in erroneously low values of exercise heart rate.

Table 5-1 **TIPS ON STARTING AN EXERCISE PROGRAM**

❑ If you have been inactive and are over age 40, check with your doctor before starting an exercise program.

❑ Take time to warm-up before exercising and take time to cool-down at the end of exercise.

❑ Wear comfortable clothing appropriate for the activity and weather.

❑ Convenient and fun exercises are easier to stick with. Make walking, stair climbing, etc., a part of daily routine.

Table 5-2 **WALKING PROGRAM**

Week	Warm-Up Slow Walk	Target Brisk Walk	Cool-Down Slow Walk	Total Time
1	5 minutes	8 minutes	5 minutes	18 minutes
2	5 minutes	10 minutes	5 minutes	20 minutes
3	5 minutes	12 minutes	5 minutes	22 minutes
4	5 minutes	14 minutes	5 minutes	24 minutes
5	5 minutes	16 minutes	5 minutes	26 minutes
6	5 minutes	18 minutes	5 minutes	28 minutes
7	5 minutes	20 minutes	5 minutes	30 minutes
8	5 minutes	22 minutes	5 minutes	32 minutes
9	5 minutes	24 minutes	5 minutes	34 minutes
10	5 minutes	26 minutes	5 minutes	36 minutes
11	5 minutes	28 minutes	5 minutes	38 minutes
12	5 minutes	30 minutes	5 minutes	40 minutes

 COUNTING YOUR EXERCISE HEART RATE

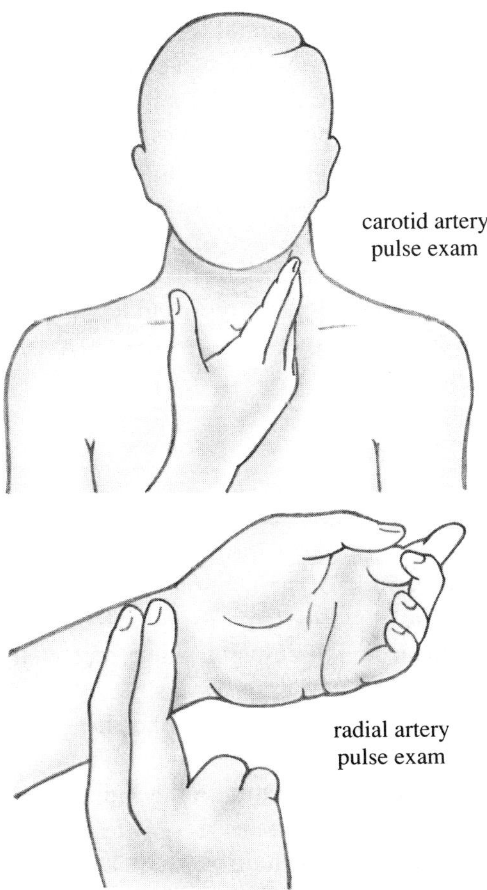

At the *moment* you stop exercise, count your carotid or radial pulse for ten seconds then multiply by six to determine your exercise heart rate.

What about sexual activity?

Almost everyone worries about having sex after heart attack, coronary bypass or coronary angioplasty. Your spouse will also be worried about sexual activity and want to be certain that this does not aggravate your heart condition in any way. These are normal feelings and emotions and should not be concern for excessive worry. Generally speaking, sexual activity can be resumed with your spouse in conjunction with resumption of your home walking program.

The separation and worry during hospitalization may make you feel uncomfortable about sex and you may want to spend additional time in other intimate contact with your spouse such as hugging and caressing. With the passage of time, however, you should be able to resume enjoyable and intimate sexual relations with your spouse. Avoid sexual activity when you are anxious or tired. If certain positions produce chest discomfort, try different positions. If angina occurs with physical exertion, your doctor may suggest taking nitroglycerin before sexual intercourse.

Know your medications

Undoubtedly, some form of medication will be prescribed at the time of hospital discharge. Understanding the reason each of these medications has been prescribed as well as their anticipated side effects will help both you and your doctor design a program of therapy best suited to your individual needs.

Digitalis preparations are used to strengthen heart muscle contraction as well as for controlling certain forms of rapid cardiac rhythm disturbance.

Diuretics, or "water pills", stimulate the kidneys to excrete excessive amounts of salt and water. This can be especially important in managing high blood pressure or fluid retention conditions such as congestive heart failure. Certain diuretics such as thiazide diuretics and loop diuretics such as furosemide (Lasix®) cause urinary losses of potassium (Table 5-3).

Your doctor may, therefore, recommend the use of potassium supplements. Other diuretics, termed "potassium sparing", may lessen this tendency toward potassium loss by combining a thiazide with a potassium- sparing compound such as triamterene or amiloride.

| Table 5-3 | **HIGH POTASSIUM FOODS** |

Fruits	*Vegetables*
Apricots	Beet greens
Apricot Nectar	Broccoli
Bananas	Brussel sprouts
Cantaloupe	Cabbage, raw
Dates	Carrots
Dried Fruit: Apricots	Dried Beans or peas
Peaches	Parsnips
Prunes	
Figs	Potatoes, white
Grapefruit juice	Pumpkin
Honeydew melon	Spinach
Nectarines	Tomatos, fresh
Oranges	Winter squash
Papaya	
Peach	
Pomegranate	
Raisins	
Strawberries	
Tangelos	
Watermelon	

Incorporating high potassium foods in the diet helps replace urinary losses associated with thiazide and furosemide diuretic therapy.

Nitroglycerin preparations are commonly used in the treatment of cardiac disease. They have multiple beneficial effects including reduction of heart work load by reducing filling pressures in the heart as well as dilating coronary arteries to improve blood supply to the heart muscle. Nitroglycerin is readily absorbed from the surface of the skin or lining of the mouth cavity and can be administered as a tablet under the tongue or as a patch applied to the skin surface. It can be prescribed in sustained release tablet form or as nitroglycerin tablets placed beneath the tongue. More recently, a nitroglycerin spray has been developed which can be given as a puff into the mouth cavity during an anginal episode.

Antiplatelet agents such as aspirin and dipyridamole (Persantine®) have an increasingly important role in the treatment of coronary artery disease and other circulatory disorders. These medications act to inhibit the first step in clot formation which is the aggregation of small circulating packets in the blood termed platelets. Antiplatelet agents are commonly used following coronary bypass graft surgery and coronary angioplasty as well as in many patients who have an established diagnosis of coronary artery disease.

Antiarrhythmic agents are used to control irregularities in cardiac rhythm. All antiarrhythmic agents entail some side effects which are usually mild in nature. The choice of an agent is specifically designed for your given type of heart rhythm disturbance and may require periodic blood tests to measure drug levels to determine if the medication is within a safe and therapeutic range. Procainamide can rarely produce a generalized inflammatory disorder termed *lupus erythematosus* which can be monitored with a blood test termed the anti-nuclear antibody. The risk of this reaction increases with higher doses of procainamide or with prolonged therapy with this agent. Your doctor will likely monitor for any signs or symptoms of lupus and may periodically obtain an anti-nuclear antibody level to determine if early lupus signs or symptoms are present. If these signs or symptoms occur, he may advise changing to an alternate antiarrhythmic agent.

Angiotensin converting enzyme inhibitors, called *ACE inhibitors*, have recently gained an important role in the treatment of heart and circulatory disorders. These agents are effective blood pressure lowering medications and also reduce the resistance to blood flow in the peripheral organs such as arms, legs and internal body organs. This significantly reduces the work load on the heart and can improve both quality of life and longevity in patients with congestive heart failure.

Calcium channel blocking agents have a variety of circulatory effects. They can be used effectively in the treatment of rapid heart rhythm from the upper chambers of the heart (atrial tachycardia) and also have an important role in the treatment of coronary artery spasm, angina pectoris, and high blood pressure.

The "beta receptor" on heart muscle tissue results in acceleration in heart rate and contracting force of the heart muscle. By inhibiting this response with beta blockers, it is often possible to reduce anginal episodes, control blood pressure, and reduce the risk of certain heart rhythm irregularities. In addition to these actions, *beta blockers* have also found a recent role in certain patients following heart attack to reduce the risk of recurrent heart attack.

Sympatholytic agents are generally used for the reduction of blood pressure. They act centrally within the brain to alter nervous system output to the heart and blood vessels, thus lowering blood pressure.

Anticoagulant therapy

Some patients with heart disease will require anticoagulant therapy with Coumadin® (warfarin). An anticoagulant is a drug which slows the clotting of blood. This may be an important component of therapy in certain patients with recent heart attack, certain patients following coronary angioplasty, and most patients with a mechanical artificial heart valve. Anticoagulants prevent new clots from forming or existing clots from further enlargement but do *not* act to dissolve existing blood clots.

Coumadin® is a very potent medication with great therapeutic potential. However, because it has the ability to alter the basic mechanism by which your body forms blood clots, there are certain inherent risks of increased bleeding while on anticoagulants. These risks can be minimized by careful observation of a laboratory test called the "prothrombin time" or "protime" for short. This test is performed by withdrawing a small sample of blood. The laboratory technician then adds several chemical ingredients and measures the time required for your blood to clot. The resulting value is measured in seconds and is often compared to a control value which represents the time necessary for normal blood to congeal (coagulate). The specific protime value necessary for treatment in your case will be determined by your physician.

A number of precautions are necessary while taking anticoagulant therapy:

1) Be certain and have your protime determined every time it is ordered by your doctor and call back to his office to determine the result. Find out what adjustment in dosage is necessary, if any.

2) Do not take any medications, especially aspirin or aspirin containing compounds, without previous approval from your doctor. Since aspirin inhibits platelet aggregation and also interferes with blood clotting, use of aspirin in conjunction with Coumadin® will increase the risk of bleeding complication. Even those medications used over the counter such as common cold remedies, antacids, laxatives or vitamins should first be cleared by your doctor.

3) Keep a record of your protime so that you can work closely in teamwork with your doctor to maintain anticoagulation within safe ranges.

4) Be certain to inform other doctors or dentists that you are taking anticoagulants before undergoing dental work or surgery. Certain changes in anticoagulant therapy will be required for some surgical procedures.

5) ***Be sure to inform your doctor if you are pregnant or planning to become pregnant since anticoagulants may be harmful to the unborn child.***

6) Report to your doctor if you are planning extended trips in order that you can make arrangements to have your protime checked while away from home.

7) Monitor closely for any obvious signs of bleeding such as
   a) prolonged bleeding from cuts, increased menstrual flow, vaginal bleeding
   b) nose bleeds, increasing bruisability or for less obvious signs of bleeding such as
      1) dark black, tarry stools
      2) red or black urine (blood in urine).

Report any of these signs or symptoms immediately to your doctor and report for a protime test.

Changes in your dietary habits or lifestyle may also change your Coumadin® requirements. Therefore, avoid binge diets. Alcohol also changes anticoagulation requirements. Alcohol should be consumed only in moderation and any change in your alcohol intake should be reported to your doctor. Since vitamin K counteracts the effects of Coumadin, avoid binges with high vitamin K foods (Table 5-4).

Anticoagulation requires a teamwork approach between patient and doctor. By careful monitoring of the protime and observing for any of the above danger signs, you can reap significant benefits from anticoagulant therapy while minimizing the inherent hazards.

Prevention of bacterial endocarditis

Certain heart and blood vessel conditions result in an increased risk of infection of these surfaces called *bacterial endocarditis*. This occurs when bacteria enter the blood stream during dental work, surgery or certain procedures.

The risk of these infections is increased in patients with abnormal heart valves whether they be leaking or obstructed heart valves. The risk is also increased in those with artificial heart valves or those with congenital defects of the heart such as atrial or ventricular septal defects. Bacterial endocarditis is a very serious condition and every effort should be made to avoid it.

The risk of endocarditis can be greatly reduced by the appropriate use of antibiotics before and after all dental work or surgical procedures. This is termed *endocarditis prophylaxis*. The American Heart Association has formulated specific antibiotic regimens and guidelines which will be familiar to your surgeon or dentist. Endocarditis prophylaxis is advised before all dental work, any major surgery, most minor surgical procedures, and certain diagnostic procedures such as examination of the bladder and some examinations of the intestinal tract.

In addition to use of antibiotics before these procedures and operations, it is important to maintain good dental hygiene. Any infections such as abscesses or skin and throat infections should be reported promptly to your doctor. Antibiotic treatment may be required in many of these instances. Signs and symptoms of heart valve infection may include fever, sweating and increased fatigability.

It is advisable to carry in your possession a list of the American Heart Association Bacterial Endocarditis Prophylaxis Recommendations and present these to your operating dentist or surgeon well in advance of any anticipated procedures. An identification bracelet indicating a need for bacterial endocarditis prophylaxis is also a wise measure.

Food	*Vitamin K* ug/100gms. (3.5 oz.)	*Food*	*Vitamin K* ug/100gms. (3.5 oz.)
Green Tea	712	Pork liver	25
Turnip greens	650	Oats	20
Broccoli	200	Green Peas	19
Lettuce	129	Whole wheat flour	17
Cabbage	125	Beef fat	15
Beef liver	92	Green beans	14
Spinach	89	Egg	8
Asparagus	57	Peach	7
Watercress	57	Ground beef	7
Bacon	46	Raisins	6
Coffee	38	Milk	3
Cheese	35	Potato	3
Butter	30	Cola	2

Returning to work

A return to work following heart attack or coronary bypass graft surgery largely depends upon the demands of your job, your overall physical condition and your type of work (Table 5-5 and Figure 5-6). This is clearly an individualized decision and is best made at approximately 4-6 weeks following check-up with your doctor. Following coronary angioplasty, many patients can return to work within one week following the procedure.

In certain circumstances, a change may be required to a different kind of work which places less burden on the heart. Effort should be made to cut down on urgent job pressures and to reduce overcrowded work schedules. Don't try to do everything yourself and avoid getting frustrated or angry over minor problems.

Most patients with heart disease can and do return to active full and pleasurable lives. Understanding your emotional response to heart disease, the need for progressive resumption in physical activity, and understanding your medications facilitates a return to an active life. Set realistic goals, and in so doing, learn to live with your heart disease.

Table 5-5 PATIENT'S DISCHARGE SUMMARY

Your Name _______________________________ Doctor's Name _______________________

Hospital Name _______________________________ Date of Hospitalization _______________

I. Diagnoses at Discharge

    1. ____

    2. ____

    3. ____

II. Procedures or Operations Performed

    1. ____ Date _______________

    2. ____ Date _______________

    3. ____ Date _______________

III. Discharge Medications

	Medication Name	Dose	When to Take
1.	__________________	__________	__________________
2.	__________________	__________	__________________
3.	__________________	__________	__________________
4.	__________________	__________	__________________
5.	__________________	__________	__________________
6.	__________________	__________	__________________

IV. Activity Instructions

____

____

____

V. Diet Instructions

____

____

VI. Special Instructions or Precautions

____

____

____

VII. Follow-up Appointments
    Doctor   Date/Time

1. _____________________ _____________________

2. _____________________ _____________________

3. _____________________ _____________________

_____________________   _____________________
  Your Signature   Doctor's Signature

CORONARY ARTERY DIAGRAM: YOUR CORONARY ARTERY BLOCKAGE AND BYPASS GRAFTS CAN BE DRAWN ON THIS DIAGRAM

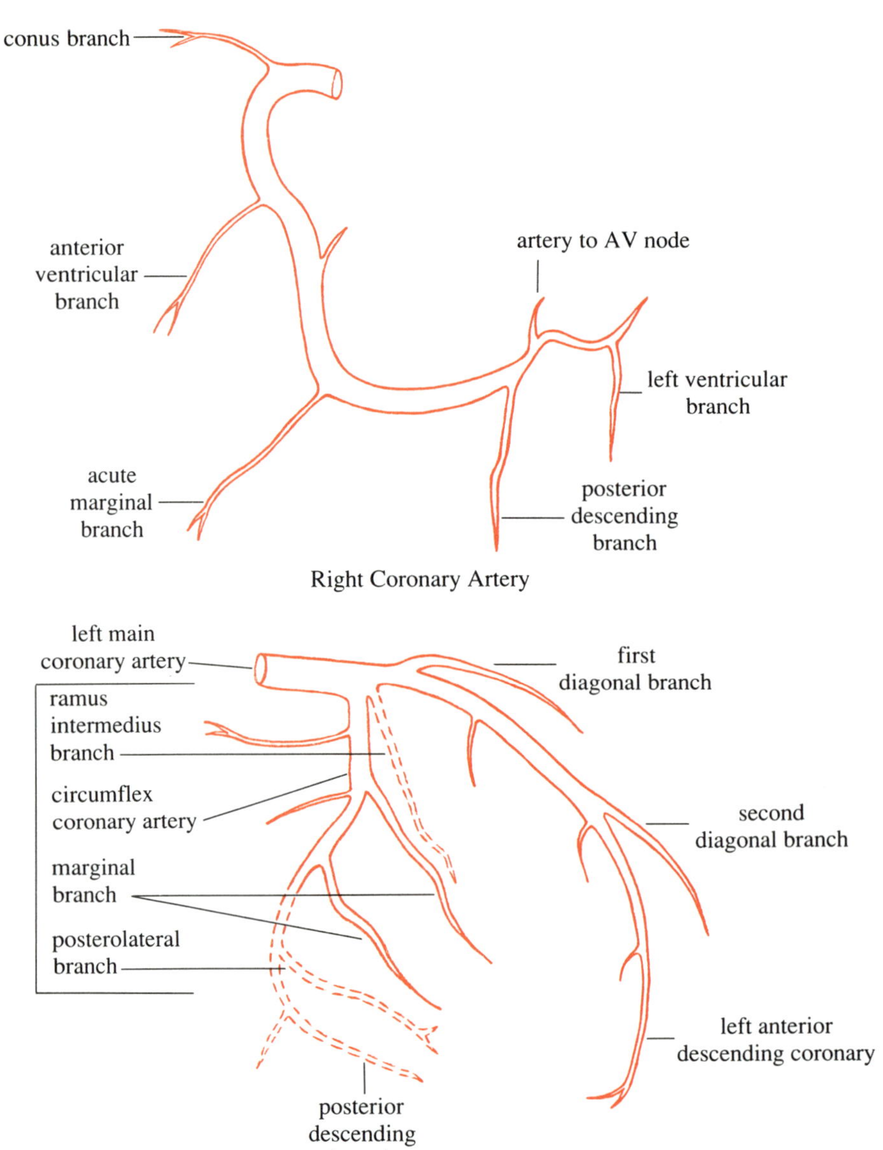

Chapter Six

Artery And Vein Disorders

Many patients with heart disease have associated atherosclerosis of arteries in the abdomen, legs and neck. Atherosclerosis in these regions can lead to stroke, leg pain with walking (claudication) or abdominal aortic aneurysm.

Carotid Artery Disease

Approximately 350,000 Americans suffer a stroke each year. Strokes occur when an area of brain is completely deprived of blood flow for a prolonged period of time. This causes irreversible damage to an area of brain and can lead to paralysis, loss of speech function or even death. Many patients who experience stroke have early warning symptoms called *transient ischemic attacks* (TIA's) (Table 6-1). These "little strokes" are due to brief episodes of impaired blood flow to the brain. They may be the result of small blood clots dislodged from diseased carotid arteries which are then carried downstream to lodge within the arteries of the eye or brain (Figure 6-1).

<hr>

Table 6-1 **WARNING SIGNS OF STROKE**

<hr>

❏ Loss or alteration of vision in one eye often described as if a shade is pulled down across the eye.

❏ Transient numbness or weakness of a body part (arm, leg, face).

❏ Momentary loss of speech or slurring of words.

❏ Transient dizziness, double vision, unusual headaches and stiffness of the neck.

These warning symptoms may present as a momentary alteration in vision such as a sudden decrease in visual acuity in one eye - often as if a shade is pulled down across the eye - or as a momentary loss or slurring of speech, as arm, leg or facial weakness, or as momentary numbness.

Not all strokes are caused by atherosclerotic disease of the carotid arteries. Blood flow to the brain can be obstructed by clots dislodged from the heart, clots dislodged from the aortic vessels, or by localized blood clot formation within the arteries of the brain itself (cerebral thrombosis). Other times, strokes can be caused by bleeding into the brain from a leaking artery (cerebral hemorrhage).

 ATHEROSCLEROTIC CAROTID ARTERY DISEASE

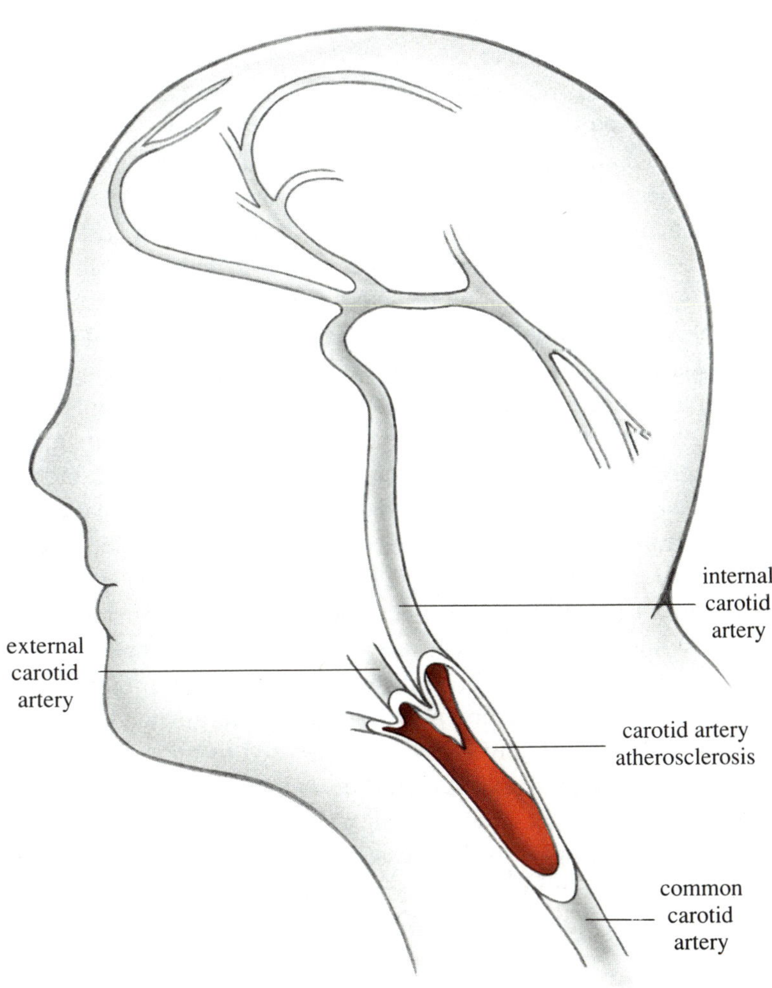

How is carotid artery disease diagnosed?

Examination of the neck with a stethoscope may reveal the presence of a high-pitched squirting noise called a *bruit*, (pronounced broo´-wee). A bruit occurs when blood attempts to rush through the narrowed carotid artery, producing a squirting noise much like that made by holding one's finger over the end of a garden hose nozzle.

However, a bruit is not always present in a diseased carotid artery, and additional information is usually required from noninvasive studies. One of the most common noninvasive studies performed today is the *Duplex Carotid Scan* (Figure 6-2). In this study, high frequency sound waves are used to take a cross-sectional picture of the carotid artery. In the neck region just below the angle of the jaw, the carotid artery divides into two branches, the internal carotid artery which supplies blood flow to the brain, and the external carotid artery which supplies blood flow to the skin and muscles of the face. Atherosclerosis commonly develops at this division, or bifurcation point. Progressive narrowing of the carotid bifurcation may result in complete carotid artery occlusion. More commonly, the atherosclerotic plaque can become "blistered" or in medical terms, *ulcerated*, forming fresh blood clot over the surface of the plaque. Fragments of these clots can detach (embolize) and lodge downstream in the brain vessels producing a transient ischemic attack (TIA) or permanent brain injury (stroke).

The severity of carotid narrowing can be determined noninvasively with ultrasound imaging. In this painless test, a gel-like substance is placed over the neck and a special ultrasound probe is moved across the neck, producing cross-sectional images of the vessel from reflections of high frequency sound waves. These reflected ultrasound waves may also be used to measure blood flow velocity within the vessel. Areas of disturbed or turbulent flow due to severe atherosclerotic narrowing can be detected by means of Doppler analysis.

If the duplex scan suggests the presence of severe carotid artery disease, oftentimes carotid angiography is performed. Under local anesthesia, a small flexible plastic catheter tube is placed in the groin artery and advanced into the carotid artery where x-ray contrast dye is injected to precisely analyze the area of carotid narrowing and to assess blood flow within the arteries of the brain.

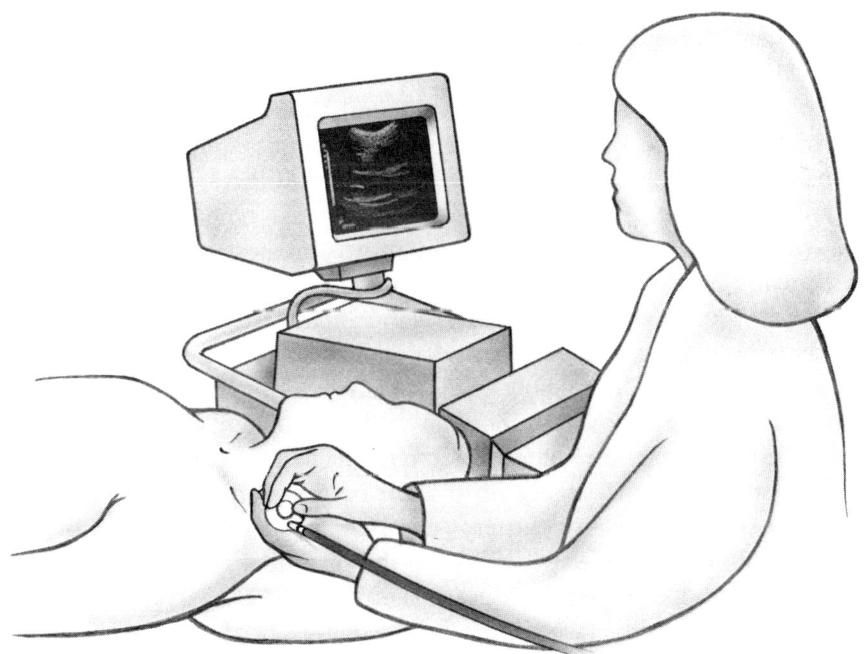

How is carotid artery disease treated?

If significant obstruction of the carotid arteries is identified, and if transient ischemic attacks are caused by this blockage, surgery is generally recommended. Surgery may also be recommended in the absence of TIA symptoms if a severe carotid obstruction is present, since the risk of TIA or stroke is increased in the presence of severe carotid obstruction. Another possible indication for surgery in a patient without TIA's is the presence of a significant carotid ulceration.

Medical therapy can also be effective for some patients with carotid artery disease. Typically, this employs the use of aspirin to reduce blood clot formation by inhibiting platelet aggregation. The aggregation of these small packets in the blood is the first step in the complex process of blood clot formation. In the Canadian Cooperative Study, aspirin therapy was demonstrated to reduce the risk of stroke and death by 19% as compared with untreated patients. The benefit of aspirin treatment was greatest for men but was not statistically significant for women. Use of more potent anticoagulants such as Coumadin® (warfarin) has also been demonstrated to be of benefit, however, the main disadvantage of long-term Coumadin® therapy remains the risk of bleeding complication in about 15% of patients.

Surgical therapy in appropriately selected patients with symptomatic carotid artery disease provides the best overall chance to reduce risk of stroke. The inherent risks of surgery itself must be weighed carefully against the anticipated benefits. Carotid artery surgery entails an inherent risk of stroke itself during or immediately following the operation as well as the risk of aggravating underlying heart disease. Therefore, the choice between medical therapy or carotid surgery is a decision which must be individualized for each patient.

How is carotid artery surgery performed?

Carotid endarterectomy is the most commonly performed surgical procedure to relieve carotid atherosclerosis (Figure 6-3). This surgery is generally performed under general anesthesia by making an incision over the carotid artery beginning beneath the angle of the jaw and extending to a level just above the collar bone (clavicle). The artery is then opened and a shunt tube

SURGICAL TECHNIQUE OF CAROTID ARTERY ENDARTERECTOMY

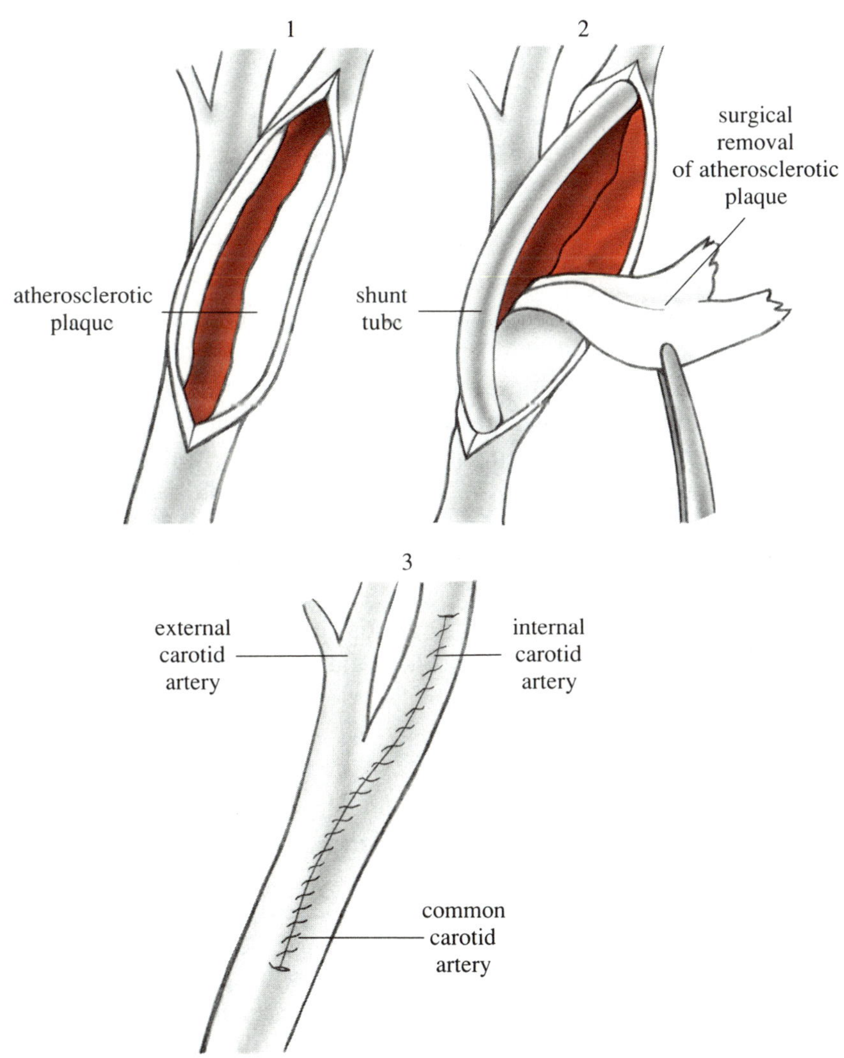

may be placed to reroute blood flow to the brain during the operation. The atherosclerotic plaque is carefully dissected off the wall of the blood vessel and removed. Once this plaque is removed, the carotid artery is sutured closed. Usually the patient is returned to the Intensive Care Unit so that blood pressure, heart rhythm, and brain function can be carefully monitored for the first 24 hours following surgery. Hospital discharge usually follows four to five days later.

Lower Extremity Artery Problems

Atherosclerosis may also narrow the arteries of the abdomen and legs. This can result in aching discomfort in the hips, thighs or calves while walking called *claudication*. Claudication is typically relieved by rest and recurs upon resumption of activity. Atherosclerosis may also weaken the wall of the aorta, causing the aorta to balloon outward producing an aortic *aneurysm*. With a progressive increase in aneurysm size, the risk of sudden rupture significantly increases. The risk of aortic aneurysm rupture increases greatly if the aneurysm becomes symptomatic (Figure 6-4). Symptoms of impending aneurysm rupture may present as low back or abdominal pain. The risk of death for symptomatic abdominal aneurysm is 30% in the first month, 74% in six months, and 80% in one year.

Progression in lower extremity arterial blockage may also result over time in such severe impairment of blood flow as to cause sores (ischemic ulceration) which fail to heal and which may result in loss of a leg or foot.

How are lower extremity artery problems and aneurysms diagnosed?

Symptoms of leg discomfort when walking which are relieved by rest may point to the presence of lower extremity peripheral artery disease. Unfortunately, many patients incorrectly assume these symptoms are the normal experiences of aging when indeed they represent claudication symptoms due to peripheral artery disease. Physical examination may reveal decreased pulses in the leg and redness of the feet when in the dependent position. Loss

REPAIR OF AN ABDOMINAL AORTIC ANEURYSM WITH A "Y" DACRON GRAFT

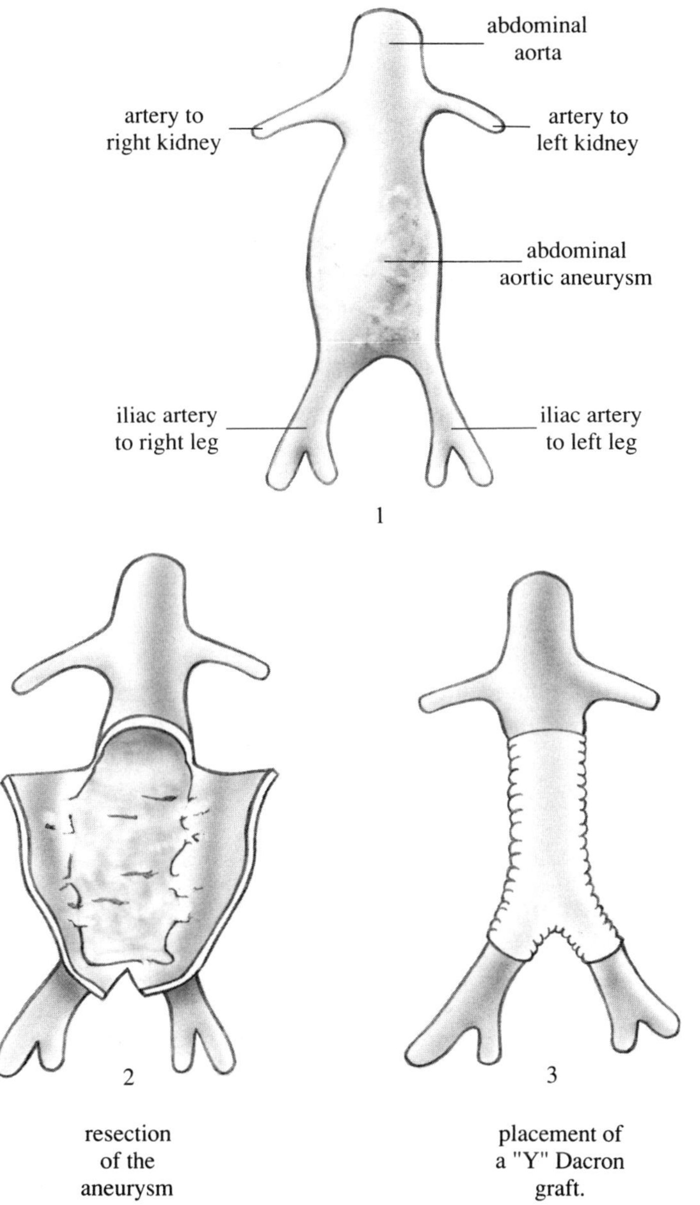

resection
of the
aneurysm

placement of
a "Y" Dacron
graft.

of hair over the lower leg and feet or excessive thickening of toenail growth may be the result of long-standing impairment of blood flow to the legs.

Noninvasive studies are extremely helpful in confirming the diagnosis of lower extremity peripheral artery disease. Application of a series of special blood pressure cuffs to the legs permits measurement of blood pressure in the thigh, calf and foot regions. Comparison of ankle blood pressures to those in the arm allows computation of an *ankle brachial index* expressed as the ankle blood pressure divided by the arm systolic blood pressure. Ankle brachial index levels are normally 1.0 or greater. Moderate to mild abnormalities of lower extremity blood flow are present when the ankle brachial is between 0.7 and 1.0. Severely abnormal blood flow to the lower extremities is present when the ankle brachial index is less than or equal to 0.5. In these circumstances, severe obstruction in multiple artery segments in the leg may be present and aching of the legs over the forefoot is often present at rest.

If an abdominal aneurysm is suspected, careful examination of the abdomen will often reveal an increase in the size and pulsatility of the abdominal aorta. The aneurysm may also be somewhat tender to gentle pressure. Abdominal ultrasound is an excellent means for measuring the size of the aneurysm cavity and for estimating the risk of aneurysm rupture. CAT scanning may also be employed to measure aneurysm size and to search for aneurysm leakage or tearing (dissection).

If severe peripheral artery disease of the legs is suspected, or if an abdominal aneurysm is discovered for which surgery is contemplated, angiography will generally be required. Angiographic injection of x-ray dye into the abdominal aorta and subsequent serial x-rays as this dye flows to the feet, allows precise evaluation of aneurysm size and extent as well as precise localization of arterial obstruction within the legs.

What treatment options are available for lower extremity artery disease?

If severe claudication symptoms are present due to obstruction of the abdominal aorta and the iliac arteries, aortobifemoral bypass grafting with synthetic Dacron graft is generally required and is often very effective for relief of symptoms. Similarly, blockage of the lower arteries in the leg can be constructed by using either the saphenous vein of the leg or a synthetic Dacron graft. Balloon angioplasty has also been employed successfully in selected obstructions of the pelvic and leg arteries. This is often a complimentary technique used in conjunction with surgical bypass (Figure 6-5). Balloon angioplasty can be performed under local anesthesia with shortened hospitalization and faster post- procedure recovery. Newer devices such as catheters designed to remove atherosclerotic debris (athrectomy catheters) or catheters with heated metal probe tips (the hot tip laser probe) also offer promise as means to open obstructed arteries without resorting to surgical bypass.

Many patients, however, do not require surgery or balloon angioplasty. Unlike the coronary arteries, the arterial circulation of the legs can often form side channels, or collaterals, around obstructed blood vessels. Formation of these collaterals can be stimulated by a regular walking program. Typically, a walking program is started by walking until claudication occurs, followed by rest and then a return to the starting point. The walk should be repeated every day and an attempt made to gradually increase the distance until a total 1-2 miles is achieved each day.

More recently the medication pentoxifylline (Trental®) has been introduced into the United States as adjunctive medical therapy for the treatment of lower extremity claudication. This medication acts to make red blood cells more deformable, thus making them more slippery, thereby reducing resistance to blood flow within narrowed arteries of the leg.

The importance of excellent foot hygiene cannot be overemphasized since complications related to foot lesions is one of the most common reasons for undertaking lower extremity arterial surgery (Table 6-2). Despite operation, amputation is required in approximately 10-20% of these cases. Therefore, prevention of foot lesions is of utmost importance. A program of daily foot care, proper footwear, regular exercise and prompt first aid treatment should be undertaken.

    TREATMENT OF LOWER EXTREMITY ARTERY BLOCKAGE BY BALLOON ANGIOPLASTY AND SURGICAL BYPASS

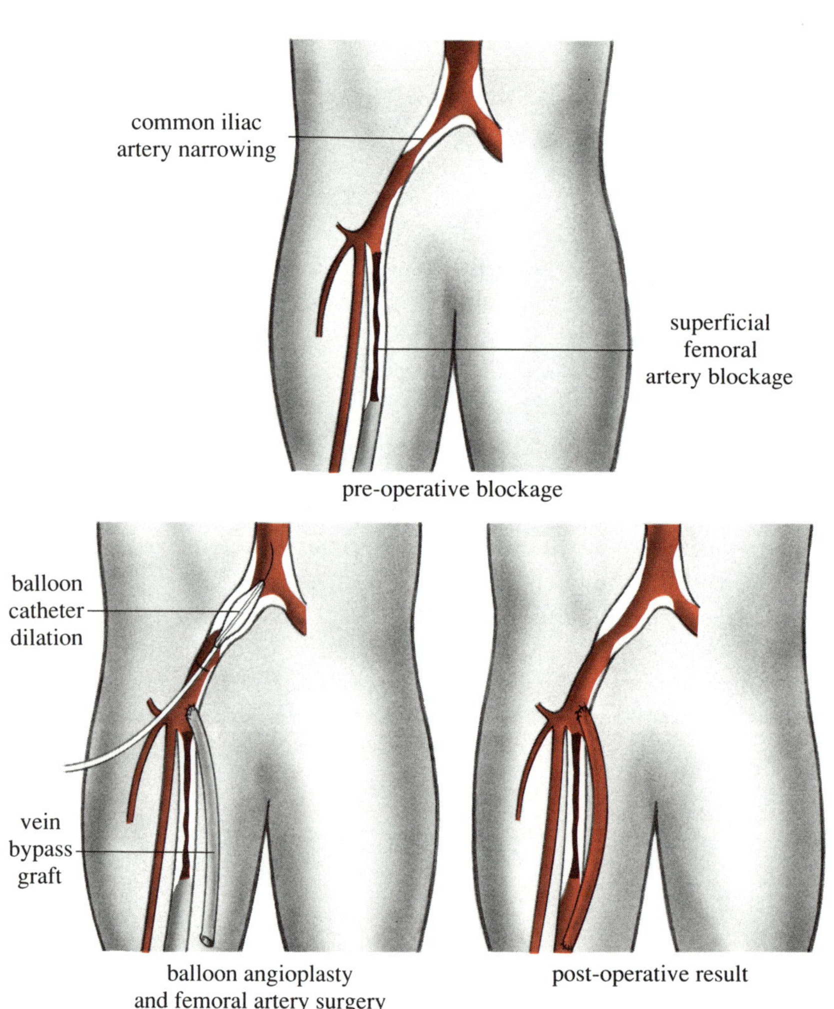

  PREVENTION OF SERIOUS FOOT PROBLEMS IN THE VASCULAR AND DIABETIC PATIENT

DO

1. Wash feet daily in lukewarm (never hot) water and mild soap, then dry thoroughly. Do not soak feet.

2. Inspect feet daily for any signs of injury, skin cracks, discoloration. Examine closely between toes and over the heels.

3. Moisturize the skin before retiring with a lanolin-based lotion.

4. Use an antifungal foot powder (Desenex®) if foot perspiration is heavy.

5. Contact your doctor or podiatrist for care of corns, calluses, and ingrown toenails.

6. Trim or cut toenails straight across with toenail clippers to avoid formation of ingrown toenails.

7. Avoid foot injuries. Place lamb's wool or absorbent gauze between toes if they are causing pressure on one another.

DO NOT

1. Go barefoot at any time.

2. Trim toenails with fingernail clippers or scissors.

3. Put talcum or baby powder in shoes.

4. Put strong chemicals or strong antiseptics (iodine) on feet.

5. Cut corns, calluses or hangnails.

LOWER EXTREMITY VEIN PROBLEMS

What are varicose veins?

Varicose veins are one of the most common vascular problems and affect approximately 15% of the adult population. Varicose veins appear as prominent distended veins easily visible under the skin of the legs. Usually they present principally a cosmetic problem, although they may cause local leg swelling (edema) and leg heaviness or aching after standing for prolonged periods of time.

Varicose veins occur when the small valves within the vein which normally prevent backflow of blood, leak and allow the vein to become swollen or varicose (Figure 6-6). Over time, increased leakage of fluid from the veins can result in hardening and thickening of overlying skin and ultimately to breakdown of the skin and formation of ulcers. However, for the vast majority of patients, varicose veins remain a cosmetic annoyance more than a threat to health.

What treatments are available for varicose veins?

Most patients with varicose veins can be treated by avoidance of aggravating factors. The following recommendations are often very helpful:

1) Avoid prolonged standing.
2) Avoid prolonged sitting.
3) Maintain body weight near ideal.
4) Avoid constricting garments.
5) Elevate the feet 10-15 minutes 3-4 times daily.
6) Apply well-fitted below-knee support stockings before ambulating in the morning.
7) Bathe or shower in the evening. This will reduce early morning lower extremity edema associated with bathing or showering in the morning.

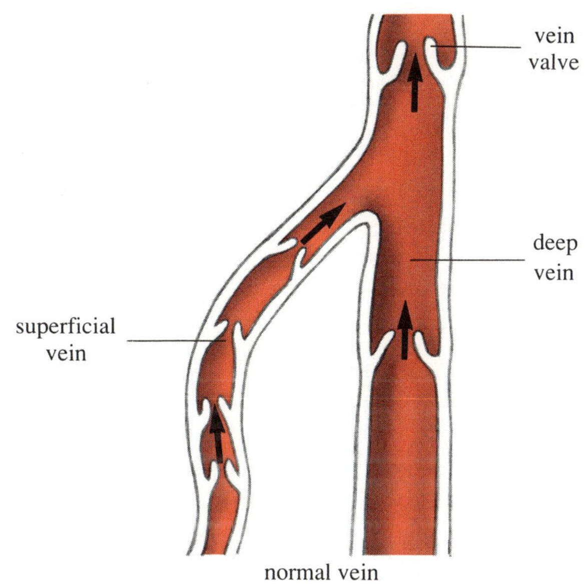

vein
valve
deep
vein
superficial
vein
normal vein

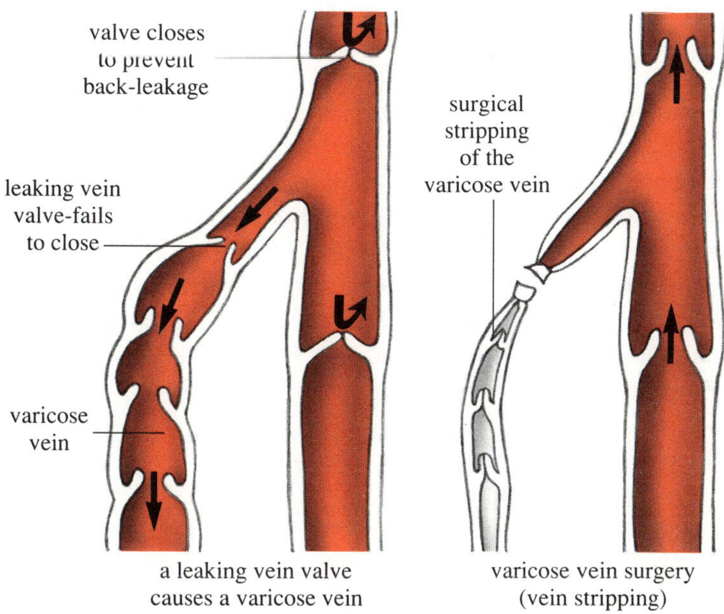

valve closes
to prevent
back-leakage
surgical
stripping
of the
varicose vein
leaking vein
valve-fails
to close
varicose
vein
a leaking vein valve
causes a varicose vein
varicose vein surgery
(vein stripping)

Should medical treatment measures fail, it may be recommended that you undergo stripping of the saphenous vein which runs along the inner aspect of the leg and thigh and stripping of the lesser saphenous vein which runs along the back of the calf.

A more difficult treatment problem is that of *deep venous insufficiency.* This occurs when the valves of the deep veins, a venous system deep within the muscles of the thighs and calves, become damaged. This results in high back pressures in the deep venous system and often leads to chronic leg edema, skin thickening and skin breakdown over the lower legs. Deep venous insufficiency is often the result of previous clot formation within the deep venous system of the leg. Treatment measures used for varicose veins may help. Skin ulceration usually requires application of a special medicated bandage called the Unna boot.

In addition to incompetent venous valves, the lower extremity veins may also develop blood clots called *venous thrombosis.* Venous thrombosis within the deep veins of the calf and knee often results eventually in deep venous insufficiency, although this may not happen until greater than ten years have passed. Therefore, any patient who has sustained deep vein thrombosis of the legs is at risk for future development of deep venous insufficiency.

The greatest risk posed by deep vein thrombosis of the thigh and pelvus is dislodgement (embolization) of deep vein clot into the venous circulation. The clot may enter the right side of the heart and lodge within a pulmonary artery, resulting in pulmonary embolization. Large pulmonary emboli often present as sudden onset of shortness of breath sometimes associated with coughing of bloody-tinged sputum. This is a potentially life-threatening problem and requires initiation of blood thinner (anticoagulant) therapy. More severe cases of pulmonary emboli have shown promising improvement when treated with clot dissolving (thrombolytic) agents such as streptokinase, urokinase, or tissue plasminogen activator (TPA).

Inflammation of the veins immediately under the skin surface, *superficial venous thrombophlebitis*, may be uncomfortable but does not directly lead to pulmonary embolization. Application of local heat, elevation of the leg, and use of anti-inflammatory medications is usually effective.

Glossary

Aneurysm - an abnormal expansion of an artery channel due to structural weakening of the artery wall.

Angina pectoris - chest discomfort produced by inadequate blood flow to the heart muscle often called angina for short. It is characterized as a squeezing or pressure-like mid chest discomfort which may radiate into the arms, neck, jaw or shoulders.

Angiogram - an x-ray picture obtained by injecting x-ray dye (contrast) into an artery usually by means of a small plastic tube (catheter).

Angioplasty - a method by which an obstructed or narrowed artery channel is opened by inflating a dilating balloon within the obstructed channel.

Angiotensin converting enzyme inhibitor (ACE inhibitor) - a medication used to inhibit the formation of angiotensin II, a potent constrictor of blood vessels within the kidney, limbs, and other body organs. ACE inhibitors can be used for treatment of high blood pressure and in treatment of congestive heart failure.

Antiarrhythmic agent - a medication used to combat irregularities in heart rhythm.

Anticoagulant - a medication used to inhibit blood clot formation within the circulation.

Antiplatelet agent - a medication used to inhibit platelet aggregation. Platelets are small, circulating packets within the blood stream which, when stimulated to aggregate, initiate the process of blood clot formation. Aspirin and dipyridamole (Persantine) are antiplatelet agents.

Aorta - the main artery leading from the heart carrying blood under high pressure to all of the body tissues.

Aortic coarctation - a congenital narrowing of the aorta which may result in high blood pressures in the arms and low blood pressure in the legs.

Aortogram - an x-ray examination of the aorta obtained by injecting x-ray dye (contrast) via a small plastic tube (catheter) placed in the aorta.

Arrhythmia - a general term which describes a disturbance in the natural rhythm of the heart.

Arteriogram - same as angiogram.

Arteriole - the smallest terminal division of the artery system.

Arteriosclerosis - same as atherosclerosis.

Atherosclerosis - hardening of the arteries produced by deposition of fatty cholesterol-rich material on the inner lining of arteries.

Atrial fibrillation - an abnormal electrical rhythm of the upper atrial heart chambers which results in loss of regular atrial contraction.

Atrial flutter - an irregularity of upper atrial heart chamber rhythm which results in rapid and ineffective contraction of the atrial chambers, usually at a rate of approximately 250 times per minute.

Atrial septal defect - a congenital abnormality in which there is a hole in the wall (septum) between the right and left atrial chambers of the heart. This results in abnormal passage of blood between the upper atrial chambers.

Atrium - a term which refers to the upper receiving chambers of the heart.

Bacterial endocarditis - infection of the heart valves with bacteria. This may result in progressive destruction in normal valve architecture and function.

Bacterial endocarditis prophylaxis - preventative antibiotics given before and immediately after dental work or surgical procedures to reduce the risk of bacterial endocarditis (valve infection) in those patients who are at increased risk for valve infection. This includes patients with significant valvular obstruction (stenosis) or valvular leakage (regurgitation), patients with most forms of congenital heart disease, or those with artificial heart valves.

Balloon pump - a short term for intra-aortic balloon pump, a device used to assist heart pumping action.

Balloon valvuloplasty - a technique by which a narrowed heart valve is stretched by inflating a balloon catheter placed across the valve.

Beta blocker - a group of heart and blood vessel medications which act to slow heart rate, reduce blood pressure, and reduce the contracting force of heart muscle. Beta blockers also stabilize certain disorders of heart rhythm.

Bradycardia - a medical term describing slow heart rate less than 55 beats per minute.

Bruit - a squirting noise produced in an artery by narrowing of the vessel usually from atherosclerotic deposit. This is much like the squirting noise produced by placing one's finger over the end of a garden hose.

Bundle branch block - a condition in which the natural transmission of electrical signals to the lower heart chambers is slowed by disease in the nerve fibers of the heart. This results in a momentary delay in contraction of a region of heart muscle and produces significant alteration in the usual EKG configuration, and therefore may limit the usefulness of the EKG for diagnosis of heart attack and angina. Bundle branch block can involve either the right (right bundle branch block) or left (left bundle branch block) conduction bundles.

cc. - an abbreviation for the metric unit of volume, cubic centimeter. 100 cubic centimeters (100 cc.) represents approximately one-tenth of a quart.

Calcium channel blocker - a group of medications (nifedipine, diltiazem, verapamil, nicardipine) which have multiple uses in treatment of angina, heart rhythm disturbance, and high blood pressure.

Capillary - the microscopic terminal junction of the circulatory system through which the arteries connect to the veins and through which the exchange of oxygen and nutrients occur into the body tissues.

Cardiac arrest - a term used to describe the cessation of normal heart rhythm or loss of blood pressure.

Cardiac catheterization - a general term which describes the passage of small plastic tubes (catheters) into the heart for the purposes of measuring pressure, injecting x-ray dye into cardiac chambers, or injection of x-ray dye into the coronary arteries or other major blood vessels.

Cardiomyopathy - a general term describing a group of disorders, the ultimate result of which is generalized injury and deterioration of heart muscle function.

Cardiopulmonary bypass machine - an artificial heart and lung machine used to pump blood and supply oxygen to the blood during coronary bypass or other cardiac surgical procedures.

Cardioversion - a means by which a disordered heart rhythm is treated by delivery of a controlled external electrical shock.

Carotid pulse - the pulsation felt in the neck by placing one's finger over the large carotid artery which runs parallel to the windpipe (trachea).

Catheter - in cardiovascular medicine, a term used to describe any hollow plastic tube inserted into an artery or vein for purposes of blood sampling, pressure measurement, injection of x-ray dye, or balloon dilation of an obstructed vessel.

Cerebrovascular accident - a general term which describes stroke due to either obstruction of a brain vessel by clot (cerebral thrombosis or cerebral embolus) or injury to brain tissue caused by bleeding from a brain artery (cerebral hemorrhage).

Cholesterol - a soft, waxy substance necessary for normal body function including the manufacture of hormones, bile acid and Vitamin D.

Claudication - aching discomfort in the legs during exercise caused by blocked arterial flow to the legs.

Collateral blood vessel - a side channel or alternate source of blood flow to a region supplied by a blocked artery.

Commissurotomy - a surgical procedure to open a scarred and narrowed heart valve performed by incising along the natural opening lines (commissures) of the heart valve.

Congestive heart failure - a condition characterized by weakening of the heart muscle.

Contrast agent - an iodine-based x-ray dye which absorbs x-rays, thus producing a silhouette picture of a blood vessel (angiogram).

Coronary artery disease - a disease caused by narrowing or obstruction of the coronary arteries due to coronary atherosclerosis (hardening of the arteries).

Coronary bypass surgery - a surgical procedure in which an artery from within the chest (internal thoracic artery or internal mammary artery) or leg vein (saphenous vein) is used to reroute blood flow around an obstructed coronary artery.

CVA - a short term for cerebrovascular accident.

Deciliter (dl) - a metric unit of volume measurement representing 100 cubic centimeters (100 cc.). The deciliter is about one-tenth of a quart.

Defibrillation - treatment of fibrillation of the ventricular chambers by application of an electrical shock to the heart.

Diabetes - a disease characterized by abnormal metabolism of blood sugar (glucose). This results from either insufficient production of the hormone insulin or an acquired insensitivity to the natural actions of insulin.

Diastole - the relaxation phase of the heart contraction cycle during which the ventricular pumping chambers fill with blood.

Dissection - a tear which develops on the inner lining of an artery.

Diuretic - a general group of cardiovascular medications which act to enhance the excretion of salt (sodium) and water via the urine.

Doppler - a means of measuring blood flow in vessels or through heart valves by reflecting high frequency sound waves off moving blood cells.

Doppler echocardiography - use of Doppler scanning to analyze blood flow through heart valves for purposes of detecting valve obstruction or valve regurgitation.

Duplex study - a term commonly used in reference to ultrasound examination of the carotid arteries in the neck.

Dysrhythmia - a general term referring to abnormalities in heart rhythm.

Echocardiogram - a cross-sectional image of the heart produced by reflections of high frequency sound waves. The echocardiogram is obtained noninvasively by application of an ultrasound transducer to the chest wall. The examination is painless.

Edema - retention of fluid in body tissues.

Ejection fraction - the proportion of blood ejected from the left ventricle with each heart beat. Typically, a normal left ventricle ejects approximately 55% or greater of the blood from its chamber with each contraction. Thus, a normal ejection fraction is approximately 55% or greater. The ejection fraction is an important overall measure of heart muscle function.

Electrocardiogram - a graphic tracing of the electrical activity of the heart muscle.

Embolus - a dislodged blood clot which travels downstream and lodges in a distant part of the circulation.

Endothelium - the inner lining membrane of arteries and veins.

Enzyme - a chemical released from body tissues such as heart muscle in response to tissue injury.

Erythrocyte - the medical term for red blood cells.

Esophagitis - inflammation or irritation of the swallowing tube (esophagus).

Essential hypertension - high blood pressure for which no underlying cause can be determined. This is the result of a "reset" in the body thermostat for blood pressure regulation.

Exercise electrocardiogram - measurement of the electrical activity of the heart in response to the stress of exercise. This study, often called a "stress test", gives important clues as to the adequacy of coronary blood flow to the heart muscle.

False negative - a negative test result in a patient who actually has the disease for which the test is performed.

False positive - a positive test result in a patient who does not have the disease for which the test is being performed.

Femoral artery - the major artery of the groin region supplying the leg. The femoral artery is typically used for arterial entry during cardiac catheterization.

Femoral vein - the major vein in the region of the groin and which drains blood from the leg back to the heart. The femoral vein is typically used for venous entry during cardiac catheterization.

Fibrillation - a severe, chaotic disorganization of heart muscle contraction resulting in loss of rhythmic contraction of the affected heart chamber. Atrial fibrillation leads to irregularity in heart rhythm whereas ventricular fibrillation results in stoppage of heart pumping action.

Gastroesophageal reflux - regurgitation of acid contents from the stomach into the swallowing tube (esophagus).

Gram - a metric unit of weight. There are approximately 28 grams in one ounce.

HDL (high density lipoprotein) - a form of blood fat which carries a small amount of cholesterol and helps carry cholesterol away from body tissues back to the liver for excretion from the body. High levels of HDL, "healthy lipoprotein", reduce the risk of atherosclerosis.

Heart attack - irreversible damage to heart muscle due to obstruction of a coronary artery.

Heart block - a slowing or "block" in the normal transmission of electrical pulses through the heart muscle. This can result in severe slowing in heart rate and may necessitate use of medication or a pacemaker to restore normal heart rhythm.

Hematoma - a collection of blood in body tissue. Following heart catheterization, this fairly common finding is the result of seepage of some blood into the tissues surrounding the artery or vein puncture site.

Hemoglobin - the organic chemical inside red blood cells responsible for carrying oxygen to the body tissues.

Heparin - a form of blood thinner (anticoagulant) administered by intravenous infusion or injection beneath the skin.

Hepatitis - inflammation of the liver.

Heterograft valve prosthesis - an artificial heart valve derived from a pig valve or the heart membrane sac of a calf heart.

Hiatal hernia - an abnormal upward pouching of stomach through the opening (hiatus) in the diaphragm muscle between the chest and abdominal cavities.

Holter monitor - a 24-hour recording of the electrocardiogram to assist in diagnosis of heart rhythm abnormalities.

Homograft valve transplantation - a technique whereby a living valve from a recently deceased person is implanted into the recipient for purposes of replacing a damaged valve.

Hypercholesterolemia - elevated blood cholesterol.

Hypertension - elevated blood pressure.

Hyperthyroidism - overactive thyroid gland function.

Hypertriglyceridemia - elevated blood triglyceride (blood fat) level.

Hypothyroidism - underactive thyroid gland function.

Innocent murmur - a form of heart murmur which is not the result of structural disease in the heart. An innocent murmur is a common finding in children and young adults simply due to rapid blood flow through the cardiac chambers.

Invasive - a general term referring to a procedure in which a body cavity or vessel must be entered for purposes of diagnostic testing or treatment.

Ischemia - a term which refers to inadequate blood flow to a region of heart muscle or other tissue.

Korotkoff sound - the sound heard by placing a stethoscope over an artery as pressure is released from an upstream blood pressure cuff.

LDH - a short term for lactic dehydrogenase, an enzyme found in abundance in heart muscle, lung, and liver.

LDL (low density lipoprotein) - a form of blood fat rich in cholesterol. LDL is principally responsible for depositing cholesterol in artery walls resulting in atherosclerosis.

Lipid - a general term describing fatty substances in the blood (cholesterol and triglyceride).

Lipoprotein - protein-coated packages in the blood that carry fat and cholesterol. LDL and HDL are lipoproteins classified based upon their weight (density).

Mechanical valve prosthesis - an artificial heart valve composed entirely of mechanical components such as stainless steel and pyrolite carbon.

mg. (milligram) - a short-hand term for milligram, a unit of metric weight. A milligram is one one-thousandth of a kilogram.

ml. (milliliter) - a unit of metric volume. A milliliter is one one-thousandth of a liter. A cc. (cubic centimeter) is the same volume as a ml. (milliliter).

Mitral annuloplasty - a surgical technique used to repair a redundant or floppy mitral valve.

Mitral valve prolapse - floppy mitral valve leaflets which bulge backward as the valve closes. This may result in mitral valve leakage.

Mixed angina - a form of angina characterized by narrowed coronary arteries and superimposed episodes of coronary artery spasm occurring at the sites of narrowing.

MUGA study - a nuclear scan used to analyze heart muscle pumping action.

Murmur - a rumbling noise in the heart heard with the stethoscope. A murmur may be the result of blood rumbling through a narrowed heart valve, regurgitating through a leaking heart valve, communicating through a hole between heart chambers, or may be a normal finding due to accelerated blood flow.

Myocardial infarction - a medical term used to describe heart muscle damage due to a blocked coronary artery.

Myocarditis - inflammation of the heart muscle usually caused by a virus infection.

Normal sinus rhythm - the term used to describe the normal sequence of heart muscle contraction in which the upper atrial chambers contract followed by rhythmic contraction of the lower ventricular chambers.

Omega-3 fatty acid (fish oil) - a kind of polyunsaturated fat found in abundance in seafood and fatty fish.

Pacemaker - an electronic device used to stimulate heart muscle contraction and maintain normal heart rhythm.

Palliative - a procedure or treatment which lessens the severity of a condition but does not result in a cure of that condition.

Palpitation - the subjective awareness of irregularity in heart beat.

Pancreatitis - inflammation of the pancreas gland in the abdomen. The pancreas is responsible for production of digestive enzymes as well as the manufacture of insulin, a hormone necessary for the regulation of sugar metabolism.

Paroxysmal atrial tachycardia (PAT) - rapid heart beat due to irregularity in rhythm of the upper atrial heart chamber.

Partial thromboplastin time (PTT) - a measure of blood clotting used to monitor heparin therapy.

Pericarditis - inflammation of the membrane sac surrounding the heart.

Pericardium - the membrane sac surrounding the heart.

Plaque - a deposit of atherosclerotic material along the wall of an artery.

Platelet - a small microscopic circulating packet in the blood which, in response to a clotting stimulus, clumps together with other platelets eventually forming a blood clot.

Polyunsaturated fat - a fat which helps reduce blood cholesterol and found in abundance in plants such as safflower, sunflower, corn and soybean oils.

Potassium - a charged particle in the blood necessary for a normal action of many organ systems including the electrical system of the heart. Abnormalities in potassium balance can result in abnormalities of heart rhythm (arrhythmia).

Premature ventricular contraction (PVC) - premature electrical discharges from the lower ventricular chambers.

Prinzmetal's angina - angina provoked by coronary artery spasm.

Proarrhythmic - an undesired effect of an antiarrhythmic medicine which results in an increase in the number and severity of irregular heart beats.

Prophylaxis - a measure taken to prevent an illness or disorder.

Prosthetic heart valve - a general term referring to an artificial heart valve.

Protime (PT) - a measure of blood clotting. The protime is typically used to monitor the anticoagulant effect of Coumadin (warfarin).

Pseudoaneurysm - a blood pocket on the outside of an artery caused by the gradual seepage of blood through the arterial puncture.

PTCA (percutaneous transluminal coronary angioplasty) - treatment of a narrowed coronary artery by dilation with a balloon catheter.

Radial pulse - the pulse felt at the wrist immediately below the base of the thumb.

Red blood cell - a blood cellular element rich in hemoglobin and responsible for carrying oxygen and carbon dioxide to and from body tissues.

Restenosis - the process by which a coronary artery or other blood vessel previously opened by balloon angioplasty renarrows due to scar tissue formation.

Rheumatic heart disease - scarring of the heart valves due to inflammation from past rheumatic fever episodes. Rheumatic fever follows infection with the streptococcus germ, the germ that causes "strep throat" and certain skin infections.

Salt - a common term for sodium chloride, or table salt.

Saphenous vein - a large vein which runs on the inner aspect of the thigh and leg and is often used as a graft during coronary bypass graft surgery.

Saturated fat - a type of fat which raises blood cholesterol more than anything else in the diet and promotes the formation of atherosclerosis. Saturated fats are found in large quantities in foods from animal products such as meat, poultry, whole milk, dairy products, milk, ice cream and cheeses. Saturated fats are also contained in some vegetable oil such as coconut, palm kernel and palm oils.

Secondary hypertension - forms of high blood pressure produced by diseases in other organs such as coarctation of the aorta, narrowed arteries to the kidney, overactive adrenal gland function (hyperaldosteronism).

SGOT - an enzyme found in abundance in heart muscle and liver cells. Elevations in SGOT may be clues to the presence of heart attack.

Sphygmomanometer - the medical term for blood pressure cuff.

Stenosis - narrowing of an artery or valve.

Stent - a wire-like mesh device placed in an artery to prop it open.

Sternum - the medical term for breastbone.

Streptokinase - a medication used to activate the clot- dissolving properties of blood.

Stress test - a shorthand term for exercise electrocardio- gram.

Sympatholytic - a general group of medications which inhibit nervous system output from the blood pressure regulating centers of the brain.

Syncope - the medical term to describe sudden loss of consciousness.

Systole - the contraction phase of the heart pumping cycle.

Systolic - pertaining to a measurement made during systole.

Tachycardia - fast heart beat. Tachycardia is generally reserved to describe heart rates in excess of 100 beats per minute.

Thallium stress test - a nuclear scan of the heart used to measure blood flow to regions of heart muscle during exercise.

Thrombolysis - a medical term describing the dissolution (lysis) of blood clot (thrombus).

Thrombus - a blood clot.

TIA - a short term for transient ischemic attack.

Tissue plasminogen activator (TPA) - a medication which activates the clot-dissolving properties of blood and whose action is localized to those sites of actual clot formation.

Transient ischemic attack (TIA) - momentary interruption of brain function due to passage of a small blood clot through a brain artery. Rather than producing permanent impairment, these stroke-like symptoms resolve over a period of several hours. TIA's may be a warning sign of impending stroke.

Triglyceride - blood fat.

Ultrasound - a high frequency form of sound wave which when reflected from body tissues can be used to create cross- sectional images of internal body structures or measure flows through vessels and heart valves.

Unsaturated fat - a kind of fat which is typically liquid at refrigerator temperature and which has a much lower risk of producing atherosclerosis than does saturated fat.

Vasodilator - a medication whose primary mode of action is to dilate arteries and/or veins. Vasodilators are commonly used in the treatment of high blood pressure.

Vasopressor - a group of medications used to constrict arteries thereby increasing blood pressure.

Vein - a portion of the circulation which carries blood back to the heart under low pressure.

Ventricle - the lower pumping chamber of the heart.

Ventricular fibrillation - cessation of heart pumping action due to chaotic electrical activity of the ventricular chambers.

Ventricular septal defect (VSD) - a hole between the right and left ventricular chambers which allows the passage of blood between right and left sides of the heart.

Ventricular tachycardia (V-tach) - a rapid heart rhythm originating from the lower ventricular cardiac chambers. Ventricular tachycardia is often a serious heart rhythm disturbance as it might result in a significant drop in blood pressure or deterioration in heart rhythm to ventricular fibrillation.

Ventriculogram - an x-ray picture of the pumping action of the ventricular chamber obtained by injecting x-ray dye via catheter into the ventricle.

Warfarin - a blood anticoagulant.

Index

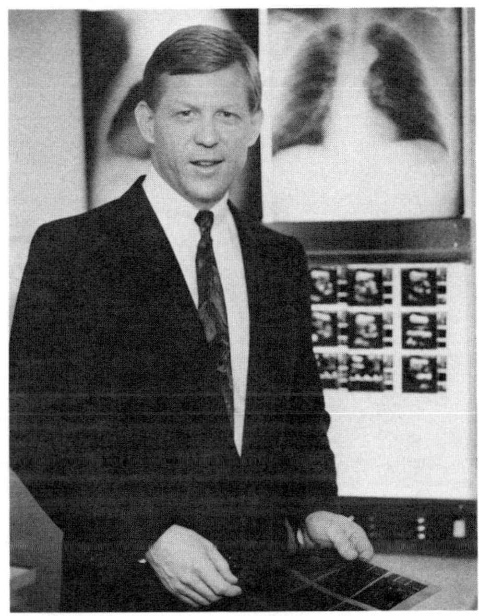

About the Author

Dr. Durand received his training in cardiology at Duke University Medical Center and is a Fellow of the American College of Cardiology (F.A.C.C.). He is board certified in both cardiology and internal medicine. Since 1982 he has been engaged in the active practice of invasive, interventional, and consultative cardiology.

NOTES

NOTES